Lecture Notes in Computer Science 11076

Commenced Publication in 1973
Founding and Former Series Editors:
Gerhard Goos, Juris Hartmanis, and Jan van Leeuwen

Editorial Board

More information about this series at http://www.springer.com/series/7412

Andrew Melbourne · Roxane Licandro
Matthew DiFranco · Paolo Rota · Melanie Gau
Martin Kampel · Rosalind Aughwane
Pim Moeskops · Ernst Schwartz · Emma Robinson
Antonios Makropoulos (Eds.)

Data Driven Treatment Response Assessment *and* Preterm, Perinatal, and Paediatric Image Analysis

First International Workshop, DATRA 2018
and Third International Workshop, PIPPI 2018
Held in Conjunction with MICCAI 2018
Granada, Spain, September 16, 2018
Proceedings

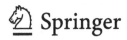

Springer

Editors
Andrew Melbourne
University College London
London, UK

Roxane Licandro
TU Wien
Vienna, Austria

and

Medical University of Vienna
Vienna, Austria

Matthew DiFranco
University of California
San Francisco, CA, USA

Paolo Rota
Italian Institute of Technology
Genoa, Italy

Melanie Gau
TU Wien
Vienna, Austria

Martin Kampel
TU Wien
Vienna, Austria

Rosalind Aughwane
University College London
London, UK

Pim Moeskops
University Medical Center Utrecht
Utrecht, The Netherlands

Ernst Schwartz
Medical University of Vienna
Vienna, Austria

Emma Robinson
King's College London
London, UK

Antonios Makropoulos
Imperial College London
London, UK

ISSN 0302-9743   ISSN 1611-3349   (electronic)
Lecture Notes in Computer Science
ISBN 978-3-030-00806-2   ISBN 978-3-030-00807-9   (eBook)
https://doi.org/10.1007/978-3-030-00807-9

Library of Congress Control Number: 2018954662

LNCS Sublibrary: SL6 – Image Processing, Computer Vision, Pattern Recognition, and Graphics

This Springer imprint is published by the registered company Springer Nature Switzerland AG
The registered company address is: Gewerbestrasse 11, 6330 Cham, Switzerland

Preface DATRA 2018

Clinical follow-up evaluation is critically important to patient care following interventions including surgical procedures, radiation therapy, or pharmaceutical treatment. As treatments become more targeted and personalized, the need arises for accurate prediction and assessment of a patient's response. Such analysis generally relies on time-related data analysis, wherein baseline and follow-up measurements are evaluated. In medical imaging, computer vision and pattern recognition approaches are being developed and adopted for such evaluations. The DATRA 2018 workshop aims at exploring pattern recognition technologies for tackling clinical issues related to the follow-up analysis of medical data with a focus on malignancy progression analysis, computer-aided models of treatment response, and anomaly detection in recovery feedback. The primary target of this workshop is to interface different backgrounds in order to outline new problems regarding the evolution of a patient's treatment response, healing, or rehabilitation. This symposium of competences can be seen as an interesting incentive to focusing on the right problems and to establishing a contact point between the medical and technical environment.

September 2018

Matthew D. DiFranco
Roxane Licandro
Paolo Rota
Melanie Gau
Martin Kampel

Organization

Organizing Committee

Matthew D. DiFranco	University of California San Francisco, USA
Roxane Licandro	TU Wien and Medical University of Vienna, Austria
Paolo Rota	Istituto Italiano di Tecnologia, Italy
Melanie Gau	TU Wien, Austria
Martin Kampel	TU Wien, Austria

Program Committee

Michael Ebner	University College London, UK
Lukas Fischer	Software Competence Center Hagenberg GmbH, Austria
Johannes Hofmanninger	Medical University of Vienna, Austria
András Jakab	University Children's Hospital Zürich, Switzerland
Bjoern Menze	TU München, Munich, Germany
Henning Müller	University of Applied Sciences Western Switzerland (HES-SO), Switzerland
Hayley Reynolds	Peter MacCallum Cancer Centre, Australia
Robert Sablatnig	TU Wien, Vienna, Austria
Marzia Antonella Scelsi	University College London, UK

Preface PIPPI 2018

The application of sophisticated analysis tools to fetal, infant, and paediatric imaging data is of interest to a substantial proportion of the MICCAI community. The main objective of this workshop is to bring together researchers in the MICCAI community to discuss the challenges of image analysis techniques as applied to the fetal and infant setting. Advanced medical image analysis allows the detailed scientific study of conditions such as prematurity and the study of both normal singleton and twin development in addition to less common conditions unique to childhood. This workshop brings together methods and experience from researchers and authors working on these younger cohorts and provides a forum for the open discussion of advanced image analysis approaches focused on the analysis of growth and development in the fetal, infant, and paediatric period.

September 2018

Andrew Melbourne
Roxane Licandro
Rosalind Aughwane
Pim Moeskops
Emma Robinson
Ernst Schwartz
Antonios Makropoulos

Organization

Organizing Committee

Andrew Melbourne   University College London, UK
Roxane Licandro   TU Wien and Medical University of Vienna, Austria
Rosalind Aughwane   University College London, UK
Pim Moeskops   Eindhoven University of Technology, The Netherlands
Ernst Schwartz   Medical University of Vienna, Austria
Emma Robinson   Imperial College London, UK
Antonius Makropoulos   Imperial College London, UK

Contents

DATRA

DeepCS: Deep Convolutional Neural Network and SVM Based Single Image Super-Resolution

Jebaveerasingh Jebadurai[✉] and J. Dinesh Peter

Department of Computer Science and Engineering,
Karunya Institute of Technology and Sciences, Coimbatore, India
jebaveerasingh.j@gmail.com

Abstract. Computer based patient monitoring systems help in keeping track of the patients' responsiveness to the treatment over the course of the treatment. Further, development of these kind of healthcare systems that require minimal or no human intervention form one of the most essential elements of smart cities. In order to make it a reality, the computer vision and machine learning techniques provide numerous ways to improve the efficiency of the automated healthcare systems. Image super-resolution (SR) has been an active area of research in the field of computer vision for the past couple of decades. The SR algorithms are offline and independent of image capturing devices making them suitable for various applications such as video surveillance, medical image analysis, remote sensing etc. This paper proposes a learning based SR algorithm for generating high resolution (HR) images from low resolution (LR) images. The proposed approach uses the fusion of deep convolutional neural network (CNN) and support vector machines (SVM) with regression for learning and reconstruction. Learning with deep neural networks exhibit better approximation and support vector machines work well in decision making. The experiments with the retinal images from RIMONE and CHASEDB have shown that the proposed approach outperforms the existing image super-resolution approaches in terms of peak signal to noise ratio (PSNR) as well as mean squared error (MSE).

Keywords: Image super-resolution · Deep learning · Deep neural networks
Rectifier linear units

1 Introduction

The development in the field of computer vision is an integral part of the development of remote health monitoring systems. Nowadays the effective application of computer vision systems directly impacts the performance of the healthcare systems. While developing a system that monitors the patients' responsiveness to the treatment, it is imperative to perform periodic analysis. Generally, the computer vision systems make use of digital images of various kinds for making decisions. The resolution of digital images play a vital role to the effectiveness of these systems. As, the high resolution images contain more useful information and higher pixel density than the low

© Springer Nature Switzerland AG 2018
A. Melbourne and R. Licandro et al. (Eds.): DATRA/PIPPI 2018, LNCS 11076, pp. 3–13, 2018.
https://doi.org/10.1007/978-3-030-00807-9_1

resolution images, they help the image analysis applications to produce more accurate results. HR images are preferred over the LR images in all the applications.

Over the years several researchers have developed image super-resolution approaches in order to improve the resolution of low resolution images. The application of SR techniques for improving has the advantages such as device independency and cost effectiveness. SR has vast application areas such as satellite imaging, medical imaging and computer vision [1–4]. The learning based approaches form end to end relationships between the low resolution patches and the high resolution patches. The learning is achieved by employing various techniques. In order to improve the quality of the high resolution image, attempts have been made by using SVM for learning and the regression of SVM to minimize the reconstruction errors. The application of neural networks has been explored by many researchers for achieving good approximation from learning [5, 6]. This paper proposes a single image super-resolution algorithm based on deep learning which will facilitate in the system that monitors patients' responsiveness to the treatment.

The remainder of this paper is organized as follows. Section 2 gives the related works. The proposed approach is explained in Sect. 3. The experimental setup and the performance evaluation are given in Sect. 4. Section 5 gives the conclusion and the future work.

2 Related Works

An elaborated study on various single image super-resolution algorithms has been carried out. The single image SR algorithms are broadly classified into reconstruction based algorithms and learning based algorithms. The reconstruction based SR algorithms focus on the elimination of aliasing artifacts from the low resolution input images but suffer from the lack of well-defined boundaries. It is also identified that, it is highly difficult to use the reconstruction based algorithms in real time applications. Further, the reconstruction based approaches fail to produce better results if the magnification factor is set over 2.

The learning based algorithms formulate the relationship between the low resolution patches of the input image and the high resolution patches of the expected output image. Various learning methods have been employed in SR algorithms. The sparse representation of images for learning is used for image super-resolution. However, it requires an additional refinement process [7, 8]. The approaches which use SVM and its regression (SVR) minimize the reconstruction error considerably. The application of SVR along with sparse coding technique produce commendable improvement in the quality of the output SR images in terms of PSNR [9, 10].

Learning with the help of neural networks (NN) has also been applied to generate high resolution results from low resolution images. Several researchers have attempted to enhance the image super-resolution process by NN based learning. Hopfield NN was used to produce SR outputs from remotely sensed images [11]. A hybrid of Probabilistic neural network and the Multi-layer perceptron was used in order to make the SR process faster [12, 13]. The usage of soft learning prior along with optical character recognition (OCR) enabled better recognition of license plates [14].

Learning with convolutional neural network produced better approximation and applied in the reconstruction of high resolution outputs [6, 15]. The deep convolutional networks with rectified linear unit (ReLU) as the activation function produce good quality outcomes [5, 16]. The application of SVM along with deep CNN improved the effectiveness of image classification [17].

This paper proposes a single image super-resolution approach that uses both the benefits of CNN as well as SVM. The major objectives of the proposed approach are 1. Generation of high resolution images from a single low resolution image, 2. Effective learning with deep CNN and 3. Effective minimization of prediction errors.

3 Proposed DCS Approach

The proposed Deep learning based single image super-resolution approach has three major layers namely patch categorization, non-linear mapping and image reconstruction. The increase in the number of layers increases the time taken for training by the neural network. Hence, the number of layers in the proposed convolutional neural network is limited to three. The proposed approach adopts the deep convolutional neural network architecture of [5]. The flow diagram of the proposed DeepCS approach is given in Fig. 1.

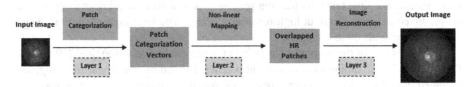

Fig. 1. Flow diagram of DeepCS approach

The patch categorization level form the patch vectors from the input low resolution images. The non-linear mapping level produces the patches of the expected high resolution image. The image reconstruction level generates the final high resolution image.

The activation functions play a vital role in the construction of any neural networks. The rectifier linear unit is used in the proposed approach as the activation function. The major advantage of using ReLU is that, it generates less number of non-zero entries which help the algorithm to learn faster. The expression explaining ReLU is given in (1), where x is the input.

$$f(x) = \max(0, x). \tag{1}$$

ReLU is better in approximation when compared to the other activation functions such as sigmoid, softmax. ReLU produces sparse representation of inputs when other activation functions generate dense representations. The size of the patch categorization filter F_1 is 1×1. Hence each and every pixel in the image will be categorized based on the outcome of ReLU activation function.

The operation using ReLU L_1 in the first layer is formulated as given in (2), where, F_1 represents filters, B_1 represents biases and $*$ represents the convolution operation. $L_1(x)$ is the value of patch categorization vector for input x.

$$L_1(x) = \max(0, F_1 * x + B_1).\tag{2}$$

The generated vectors are used as the base for non-linear mapping.

The second layer of the convolutional neural network in the proposed DeepCS approach is non-linear mapping. The results of patch categorization phase, the patch categorization vectors, are the inputs to this non-linear mapping phase. The non-linear mapping forms the predicted high resolution images.

Non-linear mapping is achieved by mapping the patch categorization vectors into the vectors of higher dimensions. The filter F_2 is used here. The non-linear mapping is done on the higher dimensional feature map rather than on the patch of the input image in order to produce the patches of higher dimensions. The dimension of filters F_2 is greater than F_1. The filters are of size 3×3 or 5×5. The non-linear mapping operation is given in expression (3).

$$L_2(x) = max(0, F_2 * L_1(x) + B_2).\tag{3}$$

Here F_2 represents filters and B_2 the biases. The increase in the number of layers also increases the time taken by training process. The results of non-linear mapping are the predicted patches of output high resolution image. The final high resolution image is constructed with these patches.

The final layer of the proposed DeepCS is the reconstruction of required HR image. The predicted overlapping high resolution patches, formed by non-linear mapping, are averaged in order to form the super-resolution output. In reconstruction, the proposed fused system exploits the advantages of support vector machines. The learned outcomes from the first two layers are used for reconstruction. The application of the regression of support vector machines (SVR) refines the image by reducing the reconstruction errors. In general, SVR is expressed as given in (4).

$$\min_{\omega, b, \xi} \tfrac{1}{2}\omega^T\omega + C\sum_{i=1}^{l}\xi_i \quad \text{s.t.}$$
$$x_i(\omega^T\phi(y_i) + b) \geq 1 - \xi_i,\tag{4}$$
$$\xi_i \geq 0, \; i = 1, \ldots, l.$$

Here x is the actual pixel for which the decision is being made, b denotes the offset parameter, l represents the number of training patches and $\phi(y_i)$ is the sparse representation of image, ω denotes the norm vector for non-linear mapping and C represents the tradeoff between the training error bounds. The sparse representation of the image is used here based on the fact that the HR image can be viewed as the sparse representation of LR patches.

Further, sparse representation for image super-resolution improves the quality of the result. Since the outcome of sparse modeling will have very few non-zero entities, it requires less time for training. Like ReLU in the first two phases, the reconstruction phase will also use very few non-zero entities. On the completion of learning with SVR, a sample high resolution result is produced. The sigmoid kernel SVR learning performs similar to a neural network with two layers. Hence, the application of sigmoid kernel SVR reduces the running time of the SR approach. The expression (5) represents sigmoid kernel where a is the magnification/scaling parameter of the input data, y denotes the vector being tested and r represents the parameter for shifting.

$$K\left(y_i, y_j\right) = \tanh\left(ay_i^T y_j + r\right). \tag{5}$$

Sigmoid kernel maps the output in a high dimensional feature space. The proposed DeepCS approach applies SVR with Bayesian decision theory in order to reduce the reconstruction errors by selecting the patch with the least error. The tradeoff between the various decisions is quantified by Bayesian decision theory by using probabilities and the associated costs or errors. According to Bayes formula, the patch which has the maximum posterior probability values will be the one that has the minimal error. It is also learned that the posterior probability of a patch and its corresponding error value are inversely proportional. The reconstruction phase results in the generation of expected high resolution image.

4 Experimental Setup and Performance Evaluation

In order to evaluate the performance, the proposed super-resolution approach was implemented and tested with several images. As the proposed approach uses the advantages of deep learning, ImageNet data set was used as learning dictionary for training the network. 24,800 sub images in ImageNet dataset are used for training the convolutional neural network. The size of training image sub size was 33 [18]. The Caffe package was used for modeling the proposed learning network.

The images taken from the datasets such as RIMONE-db-r2, RIM-ONE_database_r1, DRIONS-DB, CHASEDB1 were used as the test images. The quantitative performance of the proposed approach was evaluated in terms of MSE and PSNR. The values of MSE and PSNR were calculated using the expressions given in (6) and (7) respectively where x denotes the ground truth image of size m × n and y be the reconstructed image of same size.

MSE calculates the average of the squares of the difference between the ground truth image and the actual reconstructed result image. The PSNR and MSE are inversely proportional.

$$MSE(x, y) = \frac{1}{mn} \sum_{i=1}^{m} \sum_{j=1}^{n} \left(x_{ij} - y_{ij}\right)^2. \tag{6}$$

PSNR calculates the ratio between the maximum possible power of a signal and the power of noise that affects the quality of its representation.

$$PSNR(x, y) = 10log_{10}\left(255^2/MSE(x, y)\right). \tag{7}$$

The PSNR and MSE values were calculated for the following state of art algorithms.

- Bicubic - Bicubic Interpolation
- NE + LLE -Neighbor Embedding Locally Linear Embedding [19]
- SC + SVR - Sparse Coding with SVR SR [10]
- SLSVR - Self-Learning SR [20]
- SKSVR – Sigmoid kernel SVR [21]
- DCNN - Deep convolutional networks approach [5]
- MKSVR – Multi-kernel SVR [22]

The values of PSNR and MSE obtained after the experiments are tabulated. In tables, the values denoting the best performance for each test images are highlighted with bold letters. The MSE values require to be lesser in order to produce higher PSNR values. The PSNR values from these experiments are given in Table 1.

Table 1. PSNR values for retinal images from datasets with magnification factor 2

SR methods	NE + LLE	Bicubic	SC + SVR	SLSVR	SKSVR	DCNN	MKSVR	DeepCS
Image_002	32.30	33.98	34.14	34.20	34.31	34.53	34.64	**34.78**
Image_017	32.68	34.44	34.53	34.59	34.71	34.83	**34.91**	34.86
Image_037	30.64	32.16	32.38	32.52	32.54	32.75	32.78	**32.90**
Image_061	30.59	32.19	32.33	32.38	32.49	32.70	32.76	**32.89**
Image_081	31.41	33.12	33.19	33.25	33.36	33.58	33.64	**33.82**
IM005	41.16	41.74	43.49	43.57	43.71	43.71	**43.92**	43.87
IM102	36.96	38.16	39.05	39.12	39.25	39.50	39.50	**39.62**
IM124	38.39	39.78	40.56	40.64	40.77	41.04	41.15	**41.20**
IM144	36.59	38.10	38.67	38.71	38.87	39.12	39.24	**39.32**
IM167	39.94	41.66	42.21	42.28	42.42	42.70	**42.86**	42.82
IM256	48.44	48.64	51.19	51.28	51.30	51.78	51.80	**51.84**
IM270	42.35	43.09	44.76	44.84	44.98	45.16	45.28	**45.32**
IM293	44.60	44.70	46.13	46.21	46.77	47.37	47.41	**47.52**
IM302	43.00	43.60	45.44	45.52	45.67	45.97	45.84	**46.02**
IM319	37.31	38.90	39.43	39.50	39.63	39.68	39.92	**39.94**

From the values from Table 1, it is identified that the proposed SR approach works well for the retinal images from other globally available datasets as well. Similarly, the MSE values obtained from the experiments are tabulated in Table 2.

The PSNR values and the high resolution images that are obtained from the experiments for the retinal image 'IM319' are given in Fig. 2. It is inferred from Fig. 2 that the proposed approach generates better high resolution results in terms of PSNR as well as visual perception. The proposed approach improves the PSNR value by 2.63,

Table 2. MSE values for retinal images from datasets with magnification factor 2

SR methods	NE + LLE	Bicubic	SC + SVR	SLSVR	SKSVR	DCNN	MKSVR	DeepCS
Image_002	38.29	26.01	25.07	24.72	24.10	22.91	22.34	**21.63**
Image_017	35.08	23.39	22.91	22.60	21.98	21.38	**20.99**	21.24
Image_037	56.12	39.54	37.59	36.40	36.23	34.52	34.28	**33.35**
Image_061	56.76	39.27	38.03	37.59	36.65	34.92	34.44	**33.43**
Image_081	47.00	31.70	31.19	30.77	30.00	28.52	28.12	**26.98**
IM005	4.98	4.36	2.91	2.86	2.77	2.77	**2.64**	2.67
IM102	13.09	9.93	8.09	7.96	7.73	7.30	7.30	**7.10**
IM124	9.42	6.84	5.72	5.61	5.45	5.12	4.99	**4.93**
IM144	14.26	10.07	8.83	8.75	8.43	7.96	7.75	**7.60**
IM167	6.59	4.44	3.91	3.85	3.72	3.49	**3.37**	3.40
IM256	0.93	0.89	0.49	0.48	0.48	0.43	0.43	**0.43**
IM270	3.79	3.19	2.17	2.13	2.07	1.98	1.93	**1.91**
IM293	2.25	2.20	1.59	1.56	1.37	1.19	1.18	**1.15**
IM302	3.26	2.84	1.86	1.82	1.76	1.64	1.69	**1.63**
IM319	12.08	8.38	7.41	7.30	7.08	7.00	6.62	**6.59**

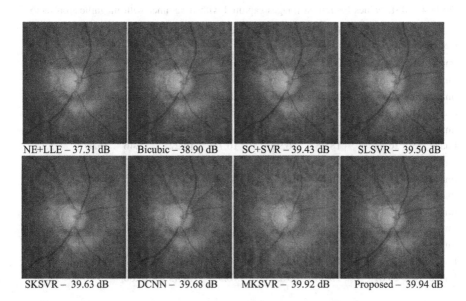

| NE+LLE – 37.31 dB | Bicubic – 38.90 dB | SC+SVR – 39.43 dB | SLSVR – 39.50 dB |
| SKSVR – 39.63 dB | DCNN – 39.68 dB | MKSVR – 39.92 dB | Proposed – 39.94 dB |

Fig. 2. SR results and PSNR values for IM319 image from RIMONE_db_r2 dataset

1.04, 0.51, 0.44, 0.31, 0.26 and 0.02 over NE + LLE, Bicubic, SC + SVR, SLSVR, SKSVR, DCNN and MKSVR approaches respectively.

Similar to the experiments with retinal images from globally available datasets, more experiments were carried out with the retinal images (100 images) captured using

Table 3. PSNR values for retinal images captured with iExaminer with magnification factor 2

SR methods	NE + LLE	Bicubic	SC + SVR	SLSVR	SKSVR	DCNN	MKSVR	DeepCS
Image_01	33.38	34.94	35.27	35.34	35.45	35.68	35.73	**35.82**
Image_02	33.68	35.27	35.59	35.68	35.75	36.04	36.00	**36.24**
Image_03	34.66	36.29	36.63	36.70	36.81	37.04	37.02	**37.12**
Image_04	34.42	36.03	36.37	36.44	36.52	36.79	36.77	**36.86**
Image_05	33.78	35.36	35.69	35.78	35.88	36.11	36.02	**36.12**
Image_06	33.93	35.51	35.84	35.90	36.03	36.24	**36.35**	36.33
Image_07	33.80	35.72	35.71	35.78	35.80	36.24	36.17	**36.38**
Image_08	34.10	36.04	36.03	36.10	36.12	36.45	36.48	**36.60**
Image_09	33.79	35.72	35.71	35.77	35.79	36.13	36.19	**36.32**
Image_10	33.95	35.88	35.87	35.94	35.96	36.29	36.33	**36.44**
Image_11	34.76	36.73	36.72	36.79	36.81	37.16	37.22	**37.30**
Image_12	34.26	35.04	36.20	36.26	36.38	**36.42**	36.36	36.40
Image_13	34.28	35.12	36.22	36.38	36.40	36.63	36.66	**36.84**
Image_14	33.87	34.69	35.77	35.95	35.97	36.20	36.24	**36.40**

Table 4. MSE values for retinal images captured with iExaminer with magnification factor 2

SR methods	NE + LLE	Bicubic	SC + SVR	SLSVR	SKSVR	DCNN	MKSVR	DeepCS
Image_01	29.86	20.85	19.32	19.01	18.54	17.58	17.38	**17.02**
Image_02	27.87	19.32	17.95	17.58	17.30	16.18	16.33	**15.46**
Image_03	22.24	15.28	14.13	13.90	13.55	12.86	12.91	**12.62**
Image_04	23.50	16.22	15.00	14.76	14.49	13.62	13.68	**13.40**
Image_05	27.23	18.93	17.54	17.18	16.79	15.93	16.26	**15.89**
Image_06	26.31	18.28	16.95	16.71	16.22	15.46	**15.07**	15.14
Image_07	27.11	17.42	17.46	17.18	17.10	15.46	15.71	**14.97**
Image_08	25.30	16.18	16.22	15.96	15.89	14.73	14.62	**14.23**
Image_09	27.17	17.42	17.46	17.22	17.14	15.85	15.63	**15.17**
Image_10	26.19	16.79	16.83	16.56	16.48	15.28	15.14	**14.76**
Image_11	21.73	13.81	13.84	13.62	13.55	12.50	12.33	**12.11**
Image_12	24.38	20.37	15.60	15.38	14.97	**14.83**	15.03	14.90
Image_13	24.27	20.00	15.53	14.97	14.90	14.13	14.03	**13.46**
Image_14	26.67	22.08	17.22	16.52	16.45	15.60	15.46	**14.90**

Welch-Allyn iExaminer, a smartphone based fundoscopy. The corresponding PSNR and MSE values are tabulated in Tables 3 and 4 respectively.

The PSNR values and the high resolution images that are obtained from the experiments for the retinal image 'Image_14' are given in Fig. 3. From Fig. 3 it is identified that the proposed approach produces better high resolution images than the state of the art approaches. The proposed approach improved the PSNR values by 2.53,

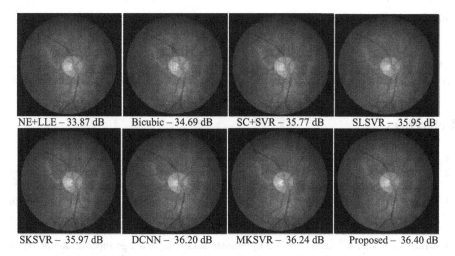

Fig. 3. SR results and PSNR values for retinal image Image_14

Table 5. Average PSNR and Average MSE values

SR methods	Average PSNR	Average MSE
NE + LLE	35.97	22.89
Bicubic	37.33	16.07
SC + SVR	37.97	14.79
SLSVR	38.05	14.52
SKSVR	38.15	14.25
DCNN	38.41	13.49
MKSVR	38.45	13.37
DeepCS	38.55	13.04

1.71, 0.63, 0.45, 0.43, 0.20 and 0.16 over NE + LLE, Bicubic, SC + SVR, SLSVR, SKSVR, DCNN and MKSVR approaches respectively. The average values of PSNR and MSE obtained from the experiments are given in Table 5. It is identified from Table 5, that the proposed approach produces better quantitative values when compared to the state of the art single image super-resolution approaches.

5   Conclusions and Future Work

A learning based single image super-resolution approach is proposed. The proposed DeepCS approach exploits the benefits of learning with convolutional neural network as well as the support vector machines. The experimental results indicated that the proposed approach produced better high resolution images than the existing approaches in terms of PSNR as well as MSE. The DeepCS approach is found to be suitable and can be used in the development of automated healthcare systems. The future works will be focused on optimizing the SR approach.

Acknowledgement. The authors thankfully acknowledge the financial support provided by The Institution of Engineers (India) for carrying out Research & Development work in this subject.

References

1. Greenspan, H.: Super-resolution in medical imaging. Comput. J. **52**(1), 43–63 (2008)
2. Wei, S., Zhou, X., Wu, W., Pu, Q., Wang, Q., Yang, X.: Medical image super-resolution by using multi-dictionary and random forest. Sustain. Cities Soc. **37**, 358–370 (2018)
3. Liang, Z., He, X., Teng, Q., Wu, D., Qing, L.: 3D MRI image super-resolution for brain combining rigid and large diffeomorphic registration. IET Image Proc. **11**(12), 1291–1301 (2017)
4. Cruz, C., Mehta, R., Katkovnik, V., Egiazarian, K.O.: Single image super-resolution based on Wiener filter in similarity domain. IEEE Trans. Image Process. **27**(3), 1376–1389 (2018)
5. Dong, C., Loy, C.C., He, K., Tang, X.: Image super-resolution using deep convolutional networks. IEEE Trans. Pattern Anal. Mach. Intell. **38**(2), 295–307 (2016)
6. He, K., Zhang, X., Ren, S., Sun, J.: Spatial pyramid pooling in deep convolutional networks for visual recognition. In: Fleet, D., Pajdla, T., Schiele, B., Tuytelaars, T. (eds.) ECCV 2014. LNCS, vol. 8691, pp. 346–361. Springer, Cham (2014). https://doi.org/10.1007/978-3-319-10578-9_23
7. Kim, K.I., Kwon, Y.: Single-image super-resolution using sparse regression and natural image prior. IEEE Trans Pattern Analysis and Machine Intelligence **32**(6), 1127–1133 (2010)
8. Yang, J., Wright, J., Huang, T.S., Ma, Y.: Image super-resolution via sparse representation. IEEE Trans. Image Process. **19**(11), 2861–2873 (2010)
9. Ni, K.S., Nguyen, T.Q.: Image superresolution using support vector regression. IEEE Trans. Image Process. **16**(6), 1596–1610 (2007)
10. Yang, M.C., Chu, C.T., Wang, Y.C.F.: Learning sparse image representation with support vector regression for single-image super-resolution. In: IEEE International Conference on Image Processing (ICIP), pp. 1973–1976 (2010)
11. Tatem, A.J., Lewis, H.G., Atkinson, P.M., Nixon, M.S.: Super-resolution target identification from remotely sensed images using a Hopfield neural network. IEEE Trans. Geosci. Remote Sens. **39**(4), 781–796 (2001)
12. Miravet, C., Rodrı, F.B.: A two-step neural-network based algorithm for fast image super-resolution. Image Vis. Comput. **25**(9), 1449–1473 (2007)
13. Miravet, C., Rodríguez, F.B.: Accurate and robust image superresolution by neural processing of local image representations. In: International Conference on Artificial Neural Networks, pp. 499–505 (2005)
14. Tian, Y., Yap, K.H., He, Y.: Vehicle license plate super-resolution using soft learning prior. Multimedia Tools Appl. **60**(3), 519–535 (2012)
15. Peyrard, C., Mamalet, F., Garcia, C.: A Comparison between multi-layer perceptrons and convolutional neural networks for text image super-resolution. In: VISAPP (1), pp. 84–91 (2015)
16. Nair, V., Hinton, G.E.: Rectified linear units improve restricted Boltzmann machines. In: Proceedings of the 27th international conference on machine learning (ICML-2010), pp. 807–814 (2010)

17. Nagi, J., Di Caro, G.A., Giusti, A., Nagi, F., Gambardella, L.M.: Convolutional neural support vector machines: hybrid visual pattern classifiers for multi-robot systems. In: the 11th IEEE International Conference on Machine Learning and Applications (ICMLA), vol. 1, pp. 27–32 (2012)

18. Deng, J., Dong, W., Socher, R., Li, L.J., Li, K., Fei-Fei, L.: ImageNet: a large-scale hierarchical image database. In IEEE Conference on Computer Vision and Pattern Recognition (CVP), pp. 248–255 (2009)

19. Chang, H., Yeung, D.Y., Xiong, Y.: Super-resolution through neighbor embedding. In: Proceedings of the 2004 IEEE Computer Society Conference on Computer Vision and Pattern Recognition (CVPR), vol. 1 (2004)

20. Yang, M.C., Wang, Y.C.F.: A self-learning approach to single image super-resolution. IEEE Trans. Multimedia **15**(3), 498–508 (2013)

21. Jebadurai, J., Peter, J.D.: SK-SVR: Sigmoid kernel support vector regression based in-scale single image super-resolution. Pattern Recogn. Lett. **94**, 144–153 (2017)

22. Jebadurai, J., Peter, J.D.: Super-resolution of retinal images using multi-kernel SVR for IoT healthcare applications. Fut. Gener. Comput. Syst. **83**, 338–346 (2018)

Automatic Segmentation of Thigh Muscle in Longitudinal 3D T1-Weighted Magnetic Resonance (MR) Images

Zihao Tang[1,2(✉)], Chenyu Wang[1,3], Phu Hoang[4], Sidong Liu[2], Weidong Cai[2], Domenic Soligo[5], Ruth Oliver[1], Michael Barnett[1,3], and Ché Fornusek[6]

[1] Sydney Neuroimaging Analysis Centre, Sydney, NSW, Australia
jack@snac.com.au
[2] School of Information Technologies, University of Sydney, Sydney, NSW, Australia
ztan1463@uni.sydney.edu.au
[3] Brain and Mind Centre, University of Sydney, Sydney, NSW, Australia
[4] Neuroscience Research Australia,
University of New South Wales, Sydney, NSW, Australia
[5] I-MED Radiology, Sydney, NSW, Australia
[6] Discipline of Exercise and Sport Science, Faculty of Medicine and Health,
University of Sydney, Sydney, NSW, Australia

Abstract. The quantification of muscle mass is important in clinical populations with chronic paralysis, cachexia, and sarcopenia. This is especially true when testing interventions which are designed to maintain or improve muscle mass. The purpose of this paper is to report on an automated method of MRI-based thigh muscle segmentation framework that minimizes longitudinal deviation by using femur segmentation as a reference in a two-phase registration. Imaging data from seven patients with severe multiple sclerosis who had undergone MRI scans at multiple time points were used to develop and validate our method. The proposed framework results in robust, automated co-registration between baseline and follow up scans, and generates a reliable thigh muscle mask that excludes intramuscular fat.

1 Introduction

Multiple sclerosis (MS) is an inflammatory disease of the central nervous system that can affect electrical conduction in axons in the brain, spinal cord, and optic nerves [3]. The clinical manifestations are partly driven by the location of focal inflammatory lesions and include paralysis/paresis, spasticity, fatigue, cognitive impairment, and sphincter dysfunction.

Regular exercise may benefit patients with MS, primarily by ameliorating deconditioning associated with disability. However, disability associated with advanced disease (Expanded Disability Status Scale (EDSS) of 7.0 or more) impedes regular exercise in this patient cohort [11,12]. Previous exercise interventions in patients with advanced MS have been short-term and largely limited

A. Melbourne and R. Licandro et al. (Eds.): DATRA/PIPPI 2018, LNCS 11076, pp. 14–21, 2018.
https://doi.org/10.1007/978-3-030-00807-9_2

to arm exercise. Recently, studies have begun to investigate the potential of electrical stimulation and other treatments to maintain leg muscle mass. To assess the efficacy of these treatments in MS, a precise and accurate quantification of limb muscle mass change is critical.

In this study, we assessed the change in longitudinal thigh muscle volume in patients with advanced MS undergoing an exercise regime based on a modified version of NMES (Neuromuscular Electrical Stimulation) cycling [5,6]. This work describes an automated segmentation pipeline to rapidly quantitate lean thigh muscle volume, and accurately estimate change over time.

Previously described methods for segmenting thigh muscle volume from MR images have utilised semi-automated approaches, including threshold algorithms and model matching techniques [2,9]. More recently, semantic segmentation has become a popular approach for solving computer vision problems; and attempts have been made to segment muscle masks from MR images with deep learning based algorithms [1]. However, these models normally do not take the intramuscular fat of subject into account. Additionally, longitudinal changes in thigh muscle ROIs (regions of interest) have been seldom studied, and most published methods [4,10,13] employ cross-sectional segmentation without indicating the method of alignment of ROIs between baseline and follow-up images.

Hence, we propose an automated segmentation framework to rapidly and accurately quantitate longitudinal change in thigh muscle volume from MR images. The framework uses a novel two-phase registration method to strictly align the relevant ROIs between baseline and follow-up; and has been evaluated in 7 subjects. Our results indicate that the proposed method achieves a consistent geometric alignment in longitudinal MR thigh images in terms of Complex Wavelet Structural Similarity Image Metric (CW-SSIM).

2   Method

The proposed automated longitudinal thigh muscle segmentation framework is shown in Fig. 1. Any number of 3D T1-weighted MR images of both left and right thighs are used as the input to generate the corresponding muscle segmentation masks. To facilitate comparative analysis, region of interest (ROI) is defined by the analyst based on the anatomical landmarks and extends from the axial slice immediately superior to the patella to the inferior border of the gluteus maximus muscle. The pipeline only requires the analyst to select these two ROI endpoints on the baseline scan.

To maintain longitudinal coherence, the femur, which remains morphologically stable over time, is segmented at each time point. A two-phase process is used to co-register follow-up to baseline images and derive follow up ROIs in the baseline space. Inhomogeneity correction, thresholding and morphological processing are then applied to generate the final thigh muscle masks. The details is described as follow.

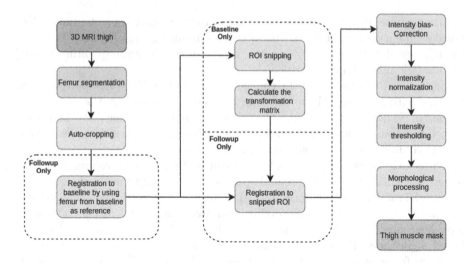

Fig. 1. Overall workflow for longitudinal thigh muscle segmentation. The raw input comprises 3D T1-weighted MR images of bilateral thighs; the pipeline outputs corresponding thigh muscle masks.

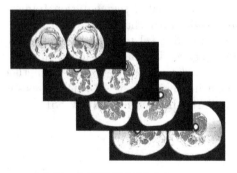

(a) Input 3D MRI thigh image

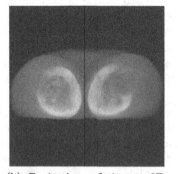

(b) Projection of input 3D MRI thigh image to axial plane

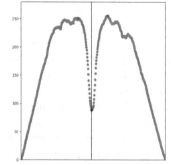

(c) Mean intensity values along sagittal plane

Fig. 2. Automated division of left and right thighs in the sagittal plane.

2.1 Cropping

The input data for each patient/scan contains both thighs, and their relative position is slightly different at each time point. Direct co-registration between baseline and follow-up will lead to an inaccurate rigid alignment result. In our pipeline, thigh muscle analysis is performed separately for left and right thighs. To achieve this, as shown in Fig. 2(b), each 3D image is firstly projected to the axial plane by averaging the voxels along the superior-inferior direction, and then further averaged to L-R line to obtain the mean intensity profile as shown in Fig. 2(c). The 3D MR thigh image is divided into left and right thigh (black line, Fig. 2(c)) in the sagittal plane, located automatically by the interpeak nadir in the associated intensity plot.

2.2 Two-Phase Registration

External deformation of muscle during scanning, or longitudinal change in muscle morphology hampers geometric alignment and accurate co-registration of baseline and follow up 3D thigh images. This is a critical step when calculating volumetric change of a ROI over time. We use a modified form of FLIRT [7] for the registration in our framework. FLIRT was originally designed for longitudinal brain registration, and is based on determining the transformation (T^*) that minimizes the intensity-based cost function:

$$T^* = arg \min_{T \in S_T} C(BL, T(FU)), \tag{1}$$

where BL and FU represent for baseline (reference) and follow-up respectively, $T(FU)$ represents for the transformed FU, S_T is the set of all affine transformations and $C(X, Y)$ is the cost function. Here we use the correlation ratio (CR) [8] as the cost function:

$$C(BL, T(FU)) = \frac{1}{Var(BL)} \sum_k \frac{n_k}{N} Var(BL_k). \tag{2}$$

When applied in this study, the default registration uses the whole thigh as the reference target. Unlike soft tissues, changes in bone morphology are negligible over the observation period; we therefore elect to define the femur as the reference target and propose a two-phase registration process: in the first phase, the transformation T_{femur}, is derived and "BL" and "FU" in Eqs. (1) and (2) are replaced with "BL_{femur}" and "FU_{femur}" respectively. T_{femur} is then applied to FU to obtain the FU_{reg}. Since we snip the ROI of the thigh along inferior-superior direction on the baseline image, the same measurement area along the thigh at follow-up is obtained by aligning the BL_{ROI} to FU_{reg}.

Figure 3 demonstrates scenarios where the use of the whole thigh as the registration reference fails to align the follow-ups with the baseline due to: (1) morphological change of muscle and fat (Fig. 3(a)); and (2) absence of distal thigh in the image (Fig. 3(b)).

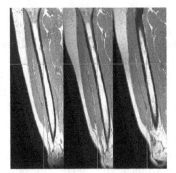 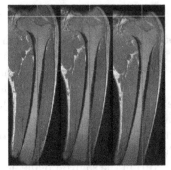

(a) A subject with massive increase of muscle volume

(b) A subject with the bottom end of femur missing

Fig. 3. Comparison of registration results in different scenarios (from left to right): baseline, registration using femur as reference and registration without using femur as reference.

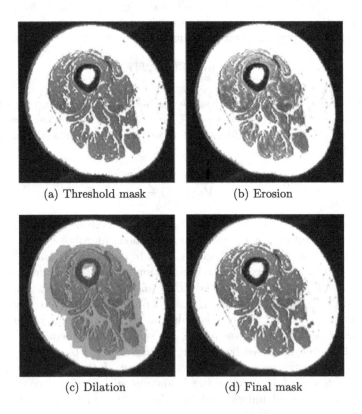

(a) Threshold mask

(b) Erosion

(c) Dilation

(d) Final mask

Fig. 4. The intermediate steps of morphological processing.

2.3   Inhomogeneity Correction and Normalization

Inherent intensity inhomogeneity in MR images requires correction before a fixed threshold is applied for the segmentation of muscle from ROIs. In our pipeline, N4 [16], an improved version of the N3 framework [15], was used. N4 achieves the result by feeding the input image iteratively into a smoothing operator which contains a B-spline approximator.

2.4   Morphological Processing

After intensity inhomogeneity-correction and normalization, a fixed intensity threshold is used to segment the thigh muscle from surrounding tissues and differentiate the muscle from the intramuscular fat. To eliminate the noisy "ring" between the outer boundary of thigh and the background, and also the border between the femur and the thigh muscle, we perform following morphological process: first performing an opening of the threshold mask then take its intersection with the original mask. The demonstration of intermediate steps is shown in Fig. 4.

3   Experimental Results

Seven participants (five females and two males) with progressive MS (median age: 55 ± 6 years old, EDSS: 7.3 ± 0.6, patients with this level of EDSS lose majority of their mobility functions) were recruited for this study from a multidisciplinary MS clinic. Participants were asked to maintain with their usual activity and exercise routines in the first 12 weeks (control period) of the study; they undertook NMES leg cycling exercises three times per week during the second 12 week study epoch. In order to obtain consistent and reliable femur imaging, patients with following scenarios were not included in the analysis: (a) inability to lie in a standard position, (b) hip replacement and (c) severe spasticity.

MRI scans (both thighs) were acquired at the time of enrolment (baseline; week 0), following the 12 week control period, and post 12 weeks of NMES training (week 24). Additionally, long-term data was acquired from two patients. In summary, 21 MRI exams (7 baseline, 7 mid-study and 7 post-NMES) were acquired on a GE Discovery MR750 Scanner with 32-channel torso coil. All subjects were scanned with a 3DT1 sequence (IRFSPGR, TE = 2.7 ms, TR = 6.5 ms, acquisition metrix = 480×480, Slice thickness = 1 mm).

For qualitative evaluation of the co-registration between baseline and follow-ups, Complex Wavelet Structural Similarity Image Metric (CW-SSIM) was computed as previously described [14]. Based on CW-SSIM score, our method yielded a higher similarity between baseline femur and femur on the co-registered follow-ups as shown in Table 1.

Table 1. Similarities between the baseline femur and femur on the co-registered follow-ups.

Subject	FLIRT	Proposed
Subject1	0.2073 ± 0.0227	0.2109 ± 0.0218
Subject2	0.2265 ± 0.0373	0.2315 ± 0.0374
Subject3	0.2303 ± 0.0392	0.2577 ± 0.0330
Subject4	0.2133 ± 0.0210	0.2165 ± 0.0201
Subject5	0.2693 ± 0.0027	0.3338 ± 0.0089
Subject6	0.2002 ± 0.0199	0.2451 ± 0.0165
Subject7	0.1145 ± 0.0497	0.1503 ± 0.0466

4   Conclusion

In this paper, we propose an automated longitudinal thigh muscle segmentation framework to calculate muscle volume change over time to assess the treatment effect. The technique can be potentially modified to sample upper arm musculature, and is ideally suited to applications requiring calculation of longitudinal changes in lean muscle mass. Femur-based co-registration minimised registration error and resulted in improved baseline to follow up image alignment, as measured by CW-SSIM. Low longitudinal measurement error and automation suggest that our technique will be suited to future inclusion in large clinical trials, both in the physical therapy and pharmacotherapy domains.

References

1. Ahmad, E., Goyal, M., McPhee, J.S., Degens, H., Yap, M.H.: Semantic segmentation of human thigh quadriceps muscle in magnetic resonance images. arXiv preprint arXiv:1801.00415 (2018)
2. Ahmad, E., Yap, M.H., Degens, H., McPhee, J.S.: Atlas-registration based image segmentation of MRI human thigh muscles in 3D space. In: Medical Imaging 2014: Image Perception, Observer Performance, and Technology Assessment, vol. 9037, p. 90371L. International Society for Optics and Photonics (2014)
3. Crayton, H.J., Rossman, H.S.: Managing the symptoms of multiple sclerosis: a multimodal approach. Clin. Ther. **28**(4), 445–460 (2006)
4. Ema, R., Wakahara, T., Yanaka, T., Kanehisa, H., Kawakami, Y.: Unique muscularity in cyclists' thigh and trunk: a cross-sectional and longitudinal study. Scand. J. Med. Sci. Sport. **26**(7), 782–793 (2016)
5. Fornusek, C., Hoang, P., Barnett, M., Oliver, R., Burns, J.: Effect of neuromuscular electrical stimulation cycling on thigh muscle mass and strength in persons with advanced multiple sclerosis. J. Neurol. Sci. **381**, 248 (2017)
6. Fornusek, C., Davis, G.M., Sinclair, P.J., Milthorpe, B.: Development of an isokinetic functional electrical stimulation cycle ergometer. Neuromodulation Technol. Neural Interface **7**(1), 56–64 (2004)

7. Jenkinson, M., Bannister, P., Brady, M., Smith, S.: Improved optimization for the robust and accurate linear registration and motion correction of brain images. Neuroimage **17**(2), 825–841 (2002)
8. Jenkinson, M., Smith, S.: A global optimisation method for robust affine registration of brain images. Med. Image Anal. **5**(2), 143–156 (2001)
9. Kemnitz, J., et al.: Validation of a 3D thigh muscle and adipose tissue segmentation method using statistical shape models. Osteoarthr. Cartil. **26**, S457–S458 (2018)
10. Kemnitz, J., Wirth, W., Eckstein, F., Culvenor, A.: Thigh muscle and adipose tissue changes during symptomatic and radiographic knee osteoarthritis progression– data from the osteoarthritis initiative. Osteoarthr. Cartil. **26**, S406 (2018)
11. Kurtzke, J.F.: Rating neurologic impairment in multiple sclerosis: an expanded disability status scale (EDSS). Neurology **33**(11), 1444 (1983)
12. Meyer-Moock, S., Feng, Y.S., Maeurer, M., Dippel, F.W., Kohlmann, T.: Systematic literature review and validity evaluation of the expanded disability status scale (EDSS) and the multiple sclerosis functional composite (MSFC) in patients with multiple sclerosis. BMC Neurol. **14**(1), 58 (2014)
13. Ruhdorfer, A., Wirth, W., Eckstein, F.: Longitudinal change in thigh muscle strength prior to and concurrent with minimum clinically important worsening or improvement in knee function: data from the osteoarthritis initiative. Arthritis Rheumatol. **68**(4), 826–836 (2016)
14. Sampat, M.P., Wang, Z., Gupta, S., Bovik, A.C., Markey, M.K.: Complex wavelet structural similarity: a new image similarity index. IEEE Trans. Image Process. **18**(11), 2385–2401 (2009)
15. Tustison, N., Gee, J.: N4ITK: Nick's N3 ITK implementation for MRI bias field correction. Insight J. **9** (2009)
16. Tustison, N.J., et al.: N4ITK: improved N3 bias correction. IEEE Trans. Med. Imaging **29**(6), 1310–1320 (2010)

Detecting Bone Lesions
in Multiple Myeloma Patients
Using Transfer Learning

Matthias Perkonigg[1]([✉]), Johannes Hofmanninger[1], Björn Menze[2],
Marc-André Weber[3], and Georg Langs[1]

[1] Computational Imaging Research Lab, Department of Biomedical Imaging
and Image-guided Therapy, Medical University of Vienna, Vienna, Austria
`matthias.perkonigg@meduniwien.ac.at`
[2] Institute of Biomedical Engineering, Image-based Biomedical Modelling,
Technical University of Munich, Munich, Germany
[3] Institute of Diagnostic and Interventional Radiology,
University Medical Center Rostock, Rostock, Germany
`https://www.cir.meduniwien.ac.at`

Abstract. The detection of bone lesions is important for the diagnosis and staging of multiple myeloma patients. The scarce availability of annotated data renders training of automated detectors challenging. Here, we present a transfer learning approach using convolutional neural networks to detect bone lesions in computed tomography imaging data. We compare different learning approaches, and demonstrate that pretraining a convolutional neural network on natural images improves detection accuracy. Also, we describe a patch extraction strategy which encodes different information into each input channel of the networks. We train and evaluate our approach on a dataset with 660 annotated bone lesions, and show how the resulting marker map high-lights lesions in computed tomography imaging data.

1 Introduction

Multiple myeloma (MM) is a cancer of plasma cells in the bone marrow. The most common symptom for MM are bone lesions. Bone lesions can be detected in computed tomography (CT) scans. An automated detection of lesions in CT scans is desirable, because it would accelerate reading images and could help during diagnosis and staging of multiple myeloma patients. The detection is difficult, and until now, no algorithms for automatic lesion detection in CT data have been developed. Deep learning approaches such as convolutional neural networks (CNN) are a promising direction for this problem. However, a difficulty arising with MM is the limited availability of annotated training data. The numbers of examples are smaller than those typically used for training CNNs, and the representation capacity suffers correspondingly.

Here, we demonstrate two approaches to perform lesion detection in MM using CNN architectures. First, we evaluate transfer learning as a means of

© Springer Nature Switzerland AG 2018
A. Melbourne and R. Licandro et al. (Eds.): DATRA/PIPPI 2018, LNCS 11076, pp. 22–30, 2018.
https://doi.org/10.1007/978-3-030-00807-9_3

improving the performance of our approach by transferring knowledge from a natural image classification task. Secondly, we explore two ways of representing visual input data for CNN training: a single channel approach, and an approach which distributes ranges of different hounsfield unit to different channels. We compare these approaches on a data set containing overall 660 annotated bone lesions.

Related Work. Convolutional neural networks [3] and transfer learning are used in medical imaging for a variety of applications. Transfer learning aims to transfer knowledge learned in a source task to improve learning in a target task [7]. Our approach uses a network pre-trained as a classifier on the natural image database ImageNet [1] (the source task) and then applies it as a detector of bone lesions (the target task). Fine-tuning on images extracted from CT scans is applied to adapt to the target task. Shin et al. describe a similar approach in [5]. They compare different architectures and learning protocols, transfer learning and random initalization, for lymph node detection and interstitial lung disease classification [5]. In [4] the authors show how convolutional neural networks can be used to reduce false positives while detecting sclerotic bone lesions in computer aided detection (CAD) tools. In the most closely related work, Xu et al. use a novel neural network architecture to detect bone lesions in multiple myeloma patients in multimodal PET/CT scans [8].

The proposed method differs from previous approaches in several aspects. It does not need a prior candidate detection stage before using the CNN [4], instead we use the CNN to detect lesions directly. Our approach operates on single 2D patches, while previous work used ensembles of neural networks and extracted multiple patches at one volume location [4,5]. Finally, we use volumes of a single modality (CT), instead of using a multimodal approach [8].

2 Method

We treat lesion detection as a classification task. We extract local image patches, and train a convolutional neural network to classify patches into *lesion* and *non-lesion*. We compare two ways of extracting image information and encoding it in image patches used by the CNN: a single channel approach, and a three channel approach. Furthermore, we compare two learning protocols to evaluate if the transfer of parameters of pre-trained models is superior to random initialization.

2.1 Extracting Image Patches

We extract a set of image patches $\mathbf{P}$ for training and testing from a set of whole body CT volumes $\{\mathbf{V}_1, \ldots, \mathbf{V}_n\}$. Due to the anisotrophy of the volumes in axial direction as well as to match the input channels of the CNN after transferring from a 2D natural image task, the image patches are extracted in 2D along the axial axes. For each volume $\mathbf{V}_i \in \{\mathbf{V}_1, \ldots, \mathbf{V}_n\}$ the center positions of all lesions

$\{\mathbf{x}_1^{l_i}, \ldots, \mathbf{x}_j^{l_i}\}$ are annotated. Additionally a bone mask $\mathbf{M}_i$ is provided for each $\mathbf{V}_i$. All patches $\mathbf{p} \in \mathbf{P}$ are extracted with a size of $15 \times 15\text{mm}$.

For each $\mathbf{V}_i$ and each lesion $\mathbf{x}_m^{l_i}$ a positive patch $\mathbf{p}_m^{p_i}$ is extracted centred around $\mathbf{x}_m^{l_i}$. $\mathbf{p}_m^{l_i}$ is augmented by random rotations and mirroring. This results in a set of positive patches $\mathbf{P}_{p_i}$ for each $\mathbf{V}_i$. A set of negative patches $\mathbf{P}_{n_i} = \{\mathbf{p}_1^{r_i}, \ldots, \mathbf{p}_m^{r_i}\}$ is extracted from $\mathbf{V}_i$ at m random positions $\mathbf{x}_m^{r_i}$ inside $\mathbf{M}_i$, with the restriction that they do not overlap with the extracted patches in $\mathbf{P}_{p_i}$. The negative patches $\mathbf{p}_m^{r_i}$ are not augmented. The final set of patches used for training and testing is given by $\mathbf{P} = \{\mathbf{P}_{p_i} \cup \mathbf{P}_{n_i}\}$ for all $i = 1 \ldots n$.

Figure 1 shows two ways of extracting a patch and representing the information for CNN training:

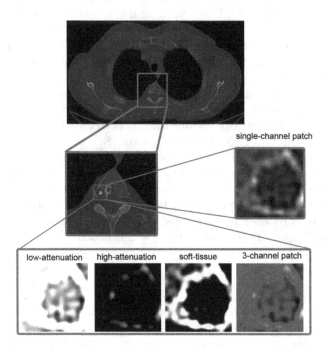

Fig. 1. Positive patch extraction: A patch is extracted along the axial axes around the center of a lesion. Single-channel patch extraction extracts gray-scale patches. 3-Channel patch extraction encodes information of a low-attenuation, high-attenuation, soft tissue window, into a combined three channel image.

1. Single channel patches: In the first approach a set of gray-scale patches $\mathbf{P}^G$ is extracted as described above. To implement transfer learning on pre-trained networks, and to match the input size of the network, the patches are rescaled to 64×64 and the same patch is fed into each of the three input channels.

2. Three channel patches: The second approach exploits the quantitative character of CT images, enabling the splitting of value ranges in a consistant manner across examples. We use three channels to encode different information extracted from the image. By this decoupling, the network can potentially find more meaningful features in different ranges corresponding to specific anatomical characteristics. We extract 3-Channel patches $\mathbf{P}^{3C}$ by assigning different ranges of Hounsfield Units (HU) to three different channels. The first channel focuses on a low-attenuation window of values smaller than 100 HU, the second on a high-attenuation window (>400 HU) and the third on a soft tissue window [100–400 HU]. The patches in $\mathbf{P}^{3C}$ are rescaled to 64×64 to match the input size of the network.

2.2   Network Architecture

We use the VGG-16 architecture [6] as a base for our network. This enables the comparison of networks trained only on our data to transfer learning using networks trained on substantially larger sets of natural images. We use $64 \times 64 \times 3$ as input size. Except the fully connected layers and the classification layer at the end of the network, the architecture remains unchanged to the original VGG-16 network. These layers are exchanged to fit the detection task resulting in a single output value. The final model used is depicted in Fig. 2. It consists of five convolutional blocks with two, respectively three convolutional layers separated by a max pooling layer with a stride of 2. In the end of the network three fully-connected layers are used. Rectified Linear Units (ReLU) are used as activation function for all hidden layers. A sigmoid activation function is used for the output unit to produce a probability value of seeing a lesion. Depending on the learning protocol used, we input different image patches to this network. The single channel patches $\mathbf{P}^{G}$ are rescaled from size 15×15 to 64×64 and the same patch is given to each channel of the input layer. The three channel patches $\mathbf{P}^{3C}$ are rescaled from $15 \times 15 \times 3$ patches to $64 \times 64 \times 3$ and each channel of the patch is used as input to one of the three input channels.

2.3   Four Models

Two different learning protocols, transfer learning and random initialization as well as two different patch extraction strategies, single channel patches and 3-channel patches, are used. For all four models trained the architecture of the network shown in Fig. 2 remains unchanged.

1. Transfer Learning: The weights of our network are transfered from pre-training a VGG-16 network on the natural image dataset ImageNet [1]. The custom fully-connected layers are initialized randomly. For the transfer learning approach the first six layers shown in Fig. 2 are frozen and the neural network is fine-tuned on $\mathbf{P}^{G}$. We fine-tune the model with stochastic gradient descent and use binary-crossentropy as loss function. The network is fine-tuned for 30 epochs. This approach will be called *TL-approach*.

2. Random Initialization: Instead of transferring from a pre-trained VGG-16 model all weights and biases are initialized randomly. The whole CNN is trained

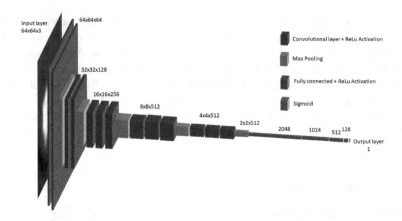

Fig. 2. The CNN architecture as used in our approach. It is based on the architecture of VGG-16 [6], the input shape and the fully connected layers at the end of the network are adapted to fit our detection task.

with stochastic gradient descent from scratch. Training is done for 40 epochs. Only $\mathbf{P}^G$ is used for training. We will call this approach *RI-approach*.

3. 3-Channel Transfer Learning approach: For this approach the transfer learning protocol is used as described above. The only difference is that we use 3-channel patches $\mathbf{P}^{3C}$ for training and evaluating the model. The approach will be denoted as *3C-TL-approach*.

4. 3-Channel Random Initialization approach: The random initialization learning protocol is used in combination with 3-channel patches $\mathbf{P}^{3C}$. The approach will be denoted as *3C-RI-approach*.

2.4 Volume Parsing

After training the network, we apply the detection to a volume of the test set $\mathbf{V}_j \in \{\mathbf{V}_1, \ldots, \mathbf{V}_t\}$, which was not part of the training process. At every position $\mathbf{x}_i^j$ within $\mathbf{M}_j$ an image patch $\mathbf{p}_i^j$ of size 15×15 millimetres along the axial axes is extracted. Depending on the model used, single channel or three channel patches are extracted, rescaled and used as input to the network. The output is a probability value $P(\mathbf{p}_i^j)$ that the patch is showing a lesion. The probabilities are visualized as a probability map of the same size as $\mathbf{V}_j$.

3 Evaluation

Data For training and evaluation a subset of the VISCERAL Detection Gold Corpus [2] is used. We use a set of 25 volumes for which manually annotated lesions and organ masks are provided. Three of those volumes, with a total of 62 lesions, are used for the evaluation of volume parsing in whole CT scans.

In the 22 CT volumes used for training and validating the CNN, a total of 598 lesions are annotated. 5938 image patches are extracted and split randomly into a training (72%), validation (10%) and test (18%) set. The training and validation set are used during the training phase of the networks. The test set is used for the evaluation of the models. Table 1 gives an overview of the dataset used for the supervised fine tuning, respectively training of the network.

Table 1. Number of samples in the dataset

	Lesion	Non-lesion
Training set	2153	2124
Validation set	299	294
Test set	538	530
	2990	2948

Evaluation on Patches. After training we evaluate the four approaches on a dataset of image patches. We measure true positives, false positives, true negatives, and false negatives. F-Score, precision and recall are computed on the test set. To evaluate if the transfer of parameters is beneficial the *TL-approach* and the *RI-approach*, respectively the *3C-TL-approach* and the *3C-RI-approach* are compared. For the evaluation of the different patch extraction strategies the results of the *TL-approach* and the *3C-TL-approach*, respectively *RI-approach* and *3C-RI-approach* are compared.

Evaluation of Volume Parsing. We parse CT volumes that were not used for training. Bone masks are used to restrict the Region of Interest (ROI) to bones. We predict a probability score for each position in the ROI and generate probability maps. Those probability maps are compared visually to evaluate the ability of the different models to detect lesions.

4 Results

Results on Image Patches. Table 2 compares different performance measures for all four models. All four approaches can classify image patches into lesion and non-lesion with high accuracy. The results show that models using transfer learning achieve a higher F-Score, and AUC, outperforming networks trained only on the CT image patches. Both approaches using transfer learning (TL-approach and 3C-TL-approach) outperform the corresponding random initialization approaches. The 3C-TL-approach has the lowest number of false negatives, which is critical as lesions should not stay undetected.

The comparison of the different patch extraction strategies demonstrates that the models trained with three channel patches performs better. The 3-channel-TL-approach (0.92) has a slightly higher F-Score than transfer learning with gray

Table 2. Comparison of detection performance measures for the four approaches: transfer learning (TL), random initialization (RI) and the 3 channel approaches (3C-TL and 3C-RI).

	Precision	Recall	F-Score	AUC
TL	0.91	0.87	0.89 ± 0.010	0.96 ± 0.006
RI	0.82	0.84	0.83 ± 0.010	0.91 ± 0.008
3C-TL	0.95	0.90	0.92 ± 0.008	0.97 ± 0.004
3C-RI	0.92	0.90	0.91 ± 0.010	0.97 ± 0.004

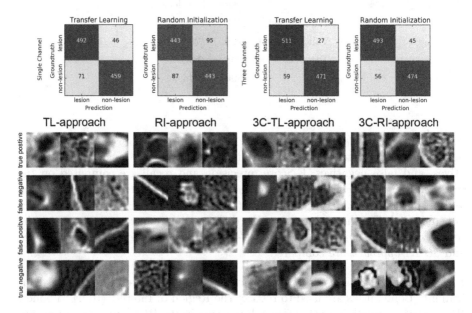

Fig. 3. Results on image patches. In the upper row confusion matrices for all four approaches are given. The lower row show examples for correct classifications and misclassifications of the networks.

scale patches (0.89). Absolute numbers and examples of true/false classifications are given in Fig. 3. The increased accuracy of the 3-channel approaches could be due to the decoupling of the different HU ranges enabling a better exploitation of the CNN architecture.

Results of Volume Parsing. Three details of probability maps for axial slices are shown in Fig. 4. The TL-approach produces smooth results with a lot of noise, while the RI-approach and the 3C-RI-approach produce more noise and sharper borders between regions classified as lesion/non-lesion. The 3C-TL approach produces the sharpest borders between regions and less noise than both RI-approaches, consistent with its higher quantitative accuracy. The qualitative analysis shows that the 3C-TL-approach outperforms the other approaches.

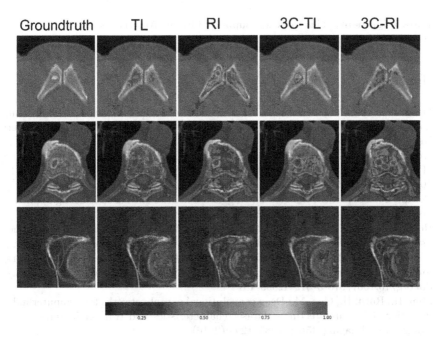

Fig. 4. Details of probability maps for detecting bone lesions in axial slices. Each row depicts the groundtruth and the detection probability of the three approaches.

The probability maps show that all approaches can detect the lesions annotated in the groundtruth. However, the false positive rate is high for all approaches with the 3C-TL approach showing the best performance. This indicates that, due to the limited number of annotated lesions in the training data, the generalization of the network is limited.

5   Conclusion

We propose an algorithm for automatic detection of bone lesions in CT data of multiple myeloma patients. We evaluated two questions: can we transfer models from natural image data to improve accuracy, and does a decoupling of HU ranges in the input representation help classification. We compared four different approaches: a CNN trained on a set of lesion and non-lesion examples of CT imaging data, a CNN pre-trained on natural images, transferred and fine tuned on the CT data, and an alternative 3-channel representation of the image data for both approaches. Results show that classification with high accuracy is possible. Transfer learning, and splitting image information into channels, both improve detection accuracy. Qualitative experiments on calculating marker maps for lesions on full volumes, show that on large volumes the suppression of false positives still needs to be improved. By providing insight the into number of lesions detected as well as their extend, the proposed method could be used in clinical context as a tool to monitor the progression of the disease.

Acknowledgement. This work was supported by the Austrian Science Fund (FWF) project number I2714-B31.

References

1. Deng, J., Dong, W., Socher, R., et al.: ImageNet: a large-scale hierarchial image database. In: Proceedings of the IEEE Conference on Computer Vision and Pattern Recognition (CVPR), pp. 248–255 (2009)
2. Krenn, M., et al.: Datasets created in VISCERAL. Cloud-Based Benchmarking of Medical Image Analysis, pp. 69–84. Springer, Cham (2017). https://doi.org/10. 1007/978-3-319-49644-3_5
3. LeCun, Y., Bottou, L., Bengio, Y., Haggner, P.: Gradient-based learning applied to document recognition. Proc. IEEE **86**(11), 2278–2324 (1998)
4. Roth, H.R., et al.: Efficient false positive reduction in computer-aided detection using convolutional neural networks and random view aggregation. In: Lu, L., Zheng, Y., Carneiro, G., Yang, L. (eds.) Deep Learning and Convolutional Neural Networks for Medical Image Computing. ACVPR, pp. 35–48. Springer, Cham (2017). https:// doi.org/10.1007/978-3-319-42999-1_3
5. Shin, H., Roth, H., Gao, M.: Deep convolutional neural networks for computer-aided detection: CNN architectures, dataset characteristics and transfer learning. IEEE Trans. Med. Imaging **35**(5), 1285–1298 (2016)
6. Simonyan, K., Zisserman, A.: Very deep convolutional networks for large-scale image recognition. In: ICLR (2015)
7. Torrey, L., Shavlik, J.: Transfer learning. In: Handbook of Research on Machine Learning Applications and Trends: Algorithms, Methods, and Techniques, 242 (2009)
8. Xu, L., et al.: W-net for whole-body bone lesion detection on ^{68}Ga-Pentixafor PET/CT imaging of multiple myeloma patients. In: Cardoso, M., et al. (eds.) CMMI/SWITCH/RAMBO -2017. LNCS, vol. 10555, pp. 23–30. Springer, Cham (2017). https://doi.org/10.1007/978-3-319-67564-0_3

Quantification of Local Metabolic Tumor Volume Changes by Registering Blended PET-CT Images for Prediction of Pathologic Tumor Response

Sadegh Riyahi[1], Wookjin Choi[1], Chia-Ju Liu[1], Saad Nadeem[1], Shan Tan[2], Hualiang Zhong[3], Wengen Chen[4], Abraham J. Wu[1], James G. Mechalakos[1], Joseph O. Deasy[1], and Wei Lu[1(✉)]

[1] Memorial Sloan Kettering Cancer Center, New York, USA
luw@mskcc.org
[2] Huazhong University of Science and Technology, Wuhan, China
[3] Henry Ford Hospital, Detroit, USA
[4] University of Maryland School of Medicine, Baltimore, USA

Abstract. Quantification of local metabolic tumor volume (MTV) changes after Chemo-radiotherapy would allow accurate tumor response evaluation. Currently, local MTV changes in esophageal (soft-tissue) cancer are measured by registering follow-up PET to baseline PET using the same transformation obtained by deformable registration of follow-up CT to baseline CT. Such approach is suboptimal because PET and CT capture fundamentally different properties (metabolic vs. anatomy) of a tumor. In this work we combined PET and CT images into a single blended PET-CT image and registered follow-up blended PET-CT image to baseline blended PET-CT image. B-spline regularized diffeomorphic registration was used to characterize the large MTV shrinkage. Jacobian of the resulting transformation was computed to measure the local MTV changes. Radiomic features (intensity and texture) were then extracted from the Jacobian map to predict pathologic tumor response. Local MTV changes calculated using blended PET-CT registration achieved the highest correlation with ground truth segmentation (R = 0.88) compared to PET-PET (R = 0.80) and CT-CT (R = 0.67) registrations. Moreover, using blended PET-CT registration, the multivariate prediction model achieved the highest accuracy with only one Jacobian co-occurrence texture feature (accuracy = 82.3%). This novel framework can replace the conventional approach that applies CT-CT transformation to the PET data for longitudinal evaluation of tumor response.

1 Introduction

Image-based quantification of tumor change after Chemo-radiotherapy (CRT) is important for evaluating treatment response and patient follow-up. Standard

© Springer Nature Switzerland AG 2018
A. Melbourne and R. Licandro et al. (Eds.): DATRA/PIPPI 2018, LNCS 11076, pp. 31–41, 2018.
https://doi.org/10.1007/978-3-030-00807-9_4

methods to assess the tumor metabolic response in Positron Emission Tomography (PET) images are qualitative and described based on a discrete categorization of reduction in Standardized Uptake Value (SUV) or Metabolic Tumor Volume (MTV) [12]. Overall volumetric difference is a global measurement that cannot characterize local non-uniform changes after the therapy [12]. For these reasons, diameter/SUV/volume based measurements are not consistently correlated to important outcomes [12]. Tensor Based Morphometry [8] exploits the gradient of Deformation Vector Field (DVF) i.e. determinant of Jacobian matrix termed Jacobian map (J), to characterize voxel-by-voxel volumetric ratio of an object before and after the transformation. $J > 1$ means local volume expansion, $J < 1$ means shrinkage and $J = 1$ denotes no change. There are many studies that utilize Jacobian map to evaluate volumetric changes. Fuentes et al. [3] used Jacobian integral (mean J×tumor volume) to measure the local volume change of irradiated whole-brain tissues in Magnetic Resonance Images and showed that the estimated change had good agreement with ground truth segmentation. In our previous work [8] we showed that Jacobian features in Computed Tomography (CT) images could predict the tumor pathologic response with high accuracy (94%) in esophageal cancer patients.

However, structural change in CT is affected by daily anatomical variations and therapy response is mostly seen in PET as metabolic activity [12]. Conventionally, metabolic tumor change is measured by deforming the follow-up tumor volume in PET and aligning it to baseline tumor volume using the transformation obtained from CT-CT Deformable Image Registration (DIR) [11]. However, PET and CT capture different properties (metabolic vs. anatomy) of a tumor, therefore applying the transformation from CT-CT registration is suboptimal. On the other hand, directly registering PET images is problematic since there are few image features to generate an accurate transformation [11].

Some attempts performed on deformable registration of PET-CT using joint maximization of intensities [4] increased the uncertainties due to heterogeneous tumor uptake in PET and different intensity distributions between two images. Additionally, deep learning methods to estimate DVF have been proposed recently. However, training deformations were generated using existing Free-Form registrations, hence the accuracy could be as good as already available algorithms [6]. Moreover, the algorithms were not tested for multi-modality registrations.

In this work, we used a linear combination of PET and CT images to generate a single grayscale blended PET-CT image using a pixel-level fusion method. Our main goal is to combine anatomic and metabolic information to improve the accuracy of multi-modality PET-CT registration for quantification of tumor change and for prediction of pathologic tumor response. The contributions are as follows:

1. Local MTV change calculated using Jacobian integral of blended PET-CT image registration achieved higher correlation with the ground truth segmentation ($R = 0.88$) compared to mono-modality PET-PET ($R = 0.80$) and CT-CT ($R = 0.67$) registrations.

2. Jacobian radiomic features extracted from blended PET-CT registration could better differentiate pathologic tumor response (AUC = 0.85) than mono-modality PET and CT Jacobian and clinical features (AUC = 0.65–0.81) with only one Jacobian co-occurrence texture feature in esophageal cancer patients.

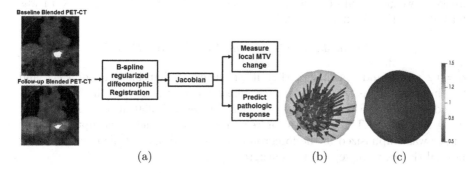

(a)   (b)   (c)

Fig. 1. (a) Main workflow of our method. Conceptual illustration of Jacobian map. (b) Larger sphere simulates MTV in the baseline image and smaller follow-up sphere illustrates shrinkage of a tumor. Converging DVF represents a volume loss and generates a Jacobian map (c) that illustrates local shrinkage (blue). (Color figure online)

2   Materials and Methods

Figure 1 shows our workflow and illustrates the concept of Jacobian map using a synthetic sphere that simulates a heterogeneous tumor shrinkage.

2.1   Dataset

This study included 61 patients with esophageal cancer who were treated with induction chemotherapy followed by CRT and surgery. All patients underwent baseline, post-induction and post-CRT PET/CT scans. Resolution for PET images was $4.0 \times 4.0 \times 4.25$ mm^3 and for CT images was $0.98 \times 0.98 \times 4.0$ mm^3. MTV on each PET-CT was segmented using a semi-automatic adaptive region-growing algorithm developed by our group [9]. Segmentations were visually reviewed and manually modified if necessary by a nuclear medicine physician. Average percentage of MTV change was $50 \pm 30.6\%$ in the cohort. Pathologic tumor response was assessed in surgical specimen and categorized into: pathologic complete responders (absence of viable tumor cells, 6 patients) and non-responders (partial response, progressive or stable disease, 55 patients). Registrations were performed between baseline and post-induction chemotherapy (follow-up) images.

2.2   Generating Blended PET-CT Images

Maximum intensity of CT images was clipped to 750 HU to eliminate the effect of high attenuation metals. PET images were resampled to CT resolution. PET and CT images were normalized to the range of [0, 1]. The normalization bounds used for CT were $(-1000, 750)$ HU and for PET, the range of tumor SUVs in our patient cohort $(0, 35)$ was used. To generate a grayscale blended PET-CT image, a weighted sum of normalized PET (nPET) and CT images (nCT) was formulated (Eq. 1) where $\alpha \in [0, 1]$:

$$Blended\ PETCT = \alpha(nCT) + (1 - \alpha)nPET \tag{1}$$

$\alpha = 0.2$ was found optimal in that it produced similar blending of PET and CT information as when the nuclear medicine physician visually fused PET (window/level = 6/3 SUV) and CT (window/level = 350/40 HU) images. By using blended PET-CT images for registration, high metabolic uptake in the tumor was emphasized in the foreground while anatomic details in surrounding normal tissues were kept in the background (Fig. 3).

2.3   Registration Methods

B-Spline Regularized Diffeomorphic Registration: To correct respiratory-induced tumor motion, we first aligned follow-up images to baseline images by rigidly registering the tumors using their center of geometry as an initial transformation. Then we deformably registered two images using a rigidity penalty term [7] to enforce the local rigidity on tumor and preserve tumor's structure while compromising on the global surrounding differences. Rigidity penalty was only applied to blended PET-CT and PET-PET registrations. Initial alignment of CT images was performed using a rigid registration. We then deployed a B-spline regularized symmetric diffeomorphic registration (BSD) [10] to characterize metabolic volume loss. A diffeomorphic registration estimates the optimized transformation, ϕ, parameterized over $t \in [0, 1]$ that maps the corresponding points between two images. ϕ is obtained by a Symmetrized Large Deformation Diffeomorphic Metric Mapping (LDDMM) algorithm that finds a geodesic solution in the space of diffeomorphism. A symmetrized LDDMM captures large intra-modality differences and guarantees inverse consistency and one-one mapping in DVF while minimizing the bias between forward and inverse transformations. By explicitly integrating the B-spline regularization term, a viscous-fluid model is formulated that fits the calculated DVF after each iteration to a B-spline object. This gives free-form elasticity to converging vectors creating a sink point that is mapped to many points in its vicinity and represents a morphological shrinkage for the regions with non-mass conserving deformations. The optimization cost function is as follows [10]:

$$c(\phi(x,t), I_b \circ I_f) = E^{MI}_{similarity}(\phi(x,1), I_b, I_f) + E^2_{geodesic}(\phi(x,0), \phi(x,1)) \tag{2}$$
$$+ \rho_{Bspline}(v(\phi(x,t)), B_k)$$

where $E^{MI}_{similarity}$ is a mutual information similarity energy, $E_{geodesic}$ is a geodesic energy function and $\rho_{Bspline}$ denotes a B-spline regularizer. The transformation $\phi(x,t)$ between baseline (I_b) and follow-up (I_f) images is characterized by the maps of the shortest path between time points $t = 0$ and $t = 1$.

$v(\phi(x,t)) = \frac{\partial \phi(x,t)}{\partial t}$ is the gradient field that defines the displacement change at any given time point. B_k is B-spline function (k spline order) applied on the gradient field. Three levels of multi-resolution registration were implemented with B-spline mesh size of 32 mm, 32 mm and 16 mm at the coarsest level for blended PET-CT, PET-PET and CT-CT registrations, respectively. The mesh size was reduced by a factor of 2 at each sequential level. The optimization step size was set to 0.15 and the number of iterations (100, 70, 40) for all modalities. We used Directly Modified Free Form Deformation optimization scheme [10] that was robust to different parameters and all the registrations were performed in a cropped region 5 cm surrounding the MTV.

Registration Evaluation Methods: We considered MTV change measured by the semi-automatic segmentation with physician modification as the ground truth to compare against Jacobian integral for registration evaluation. Correlation and percentage of difference between MTV changes calculated by Jacobian integral and by semi-automatic segmentation (ground-truth) were first assessed. Dice Similarity Coefficient (DSC) was also calculated between baseline MTV and deformed follow-up MTV. We compared BSD results with a Free-Form Deformation Registration algorithm (FFD) regularized with bending energy [5]. The blended PET-CT, PET-PET and CT-CT registrations were separately performed using these two algorithms.

Optimal Registration Parameter Estimation: (i) Regularization mesh size (σ) and (ii) optimization step size (γ) were the most sensitive parameters. We experimentally studied the influence of different $\sigma = 16, 32, 64, 128$ mm and $\gamma = 0.1, 0.15, 0.2, 0.25$ on registration and Jacobian map. The registration results were used as a quantitative benchmark to find the optimal trade-off between the parameters. A parameter set that resulted in the best DSC and the highest correlation between Jacobian integral and segmentation was chosen as the optimal parameters.

2.4   Jacobian Features for Prediction of Tumor Response

We extracted 56 radiomic features quantifying the intensity and texture [13] of a tumor in the Jacobian map. The Jacobian features quantified the spatial patterns of tumor volumetric change. The importance of features in predicting pathologic tumor response was evaluated by both univariate and multivariate analysis. In univariate analysis, p-value and Area Under the Receiver Operating Characteristic Curve (AUC) for each feature was calculated using Wilcoxon rank sum test. In multi-variate analysis, firstly distinctive features were identified using hierarchical clustering [2]. A Random Forest model (RF) was then constructed (200 trees) with features chosen by a Least Absolute Shrinkage and Selection Operator (LASSO) feature selection. All distinctive features were fed to the RF classifier in a manner of a 10-fold cross-validation (CV). Within each fold, LASSO was applied to select the ten most important features. We repeated the 10-fold CV ten times to obtain the model accuracy (10×10-fold CV).

3 Results and Discussion

3.1 Quantitative Registration Evaluation

A combination of $\sigma = 32$ mm (blended PET-CT), 32 mm (PET-PET), 16 mm (CT-CT) and $\gamma = 0.15$ achieved the best DSC and the highest correlation hence were selected as the optimal registration parameters. Larger mesh size in blended PET-CT and PET-PET registrations compared to CT-CT registration produced a more regularized and smoothed DVF to compensate the local irregular deformations due to non-uniform metabolic uptakes and lack of corresponding points in PET. Figure 2 shows scatter plots with least square regression line (solid red) between MTV change calculated by Jacobian integral and the ground truth segmentation for (a) blended PET-CT, (b) PET-PET and (c) CT-CT BSD registrations with goodness of fit (r^2) values. Blended PET-CT registration showed the highest r^2 and captured the greatest range of deformations in tumor, compared to PET-PET and CT-CT registrations. Table 1 shows correlation coefficients and average percentage of difference between Jacobian integral and segmentation using BSD and FFD for each modality.

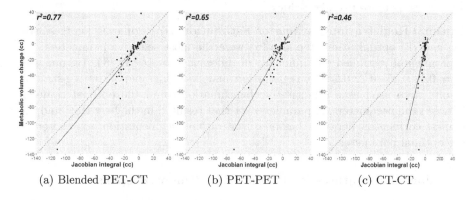

(a) Blended PET-CT   (b) PET-PET   (c) CT-CT

Fig. 2. Scatter plot showing correlation between MTV change calculated by Jacobian integral and ground truth segmentation for (a) blended PET-CT, (b) PET-PET and (c) CT-CT BSD registrations. Dashed blue line is identity line. (Color figure online)

Mean±stdev DSC are also presented in Table 1. Blended PET-CT registration showed higher DSC with less variation among the cohort. Using a blended PET-CT registration, DVF in and near the tumor region was driven by the metabolic changes while DVF outside the tumor region was driven by the

Table 1. Registration results using the optimal parameters comparing correlation and average percentage difference between MTV change estimated by Jacobian integral and segmentation.

Registration	Correlation	% Difference	DSC	Quantified changes
Segmentation	-	-	-	50%
PET-CT BSD	0.88	7.8%	0.73±0.08	42%
PET BSD	0.80	14.1%	0.66±0.13	28.6%
CT BSD	0.67	31.6%	0.69±0.16	7.6%
PET-CT FFD	0.77	18.6%	0.71±0.13	22%
PET FFD	0.74	25.1%	0.60±0.14	17.4%
CT FFD	0.32	28.4%	0.69±0.16	19.6%

anatomical structures surrounding the tumor. The blended PET-CT registration benefited by leveraging prominent image features from both PET and CT simultaneously, hence, achieving higher DSC and more accurate estimation of MTV change.

3.2 Residual Tumor versus Non-residual Tumor Cases

Figure 3 shows blended PET-CT images of 3 heterogeneous tumor cases. Tumor shrinkage calculated by blended PET-CT, PET-PET and CT-CT registrations are illustrated using DVF and Jacobian map for each case (Top, Middle and Bottom). Qualitatively, using blended PET-CT image registration, vectors converged from the boundary toward the center of baseline and follow-up MTVs (green and blue volume), generated a sink point in the center where Jacobian was much smaller than 1 (shown in blue in Jacobian map), indicating a large shrinkage. Using PET-PET registration, due to lack of image features, the registration couldn't accurately find the corresponding points and DVF only converged in the tumor boundary. For CT-CT registration, due to smaller structural change and uniform intensity in soft tissue, DVF magnitude was small and Jacobian map mostly showed no volume change. The percentage of tumor shrinkage calculated by semi-automatic segmentation (ground-truth) is listed in Table 2 for each case (Top, Middle and Bottom). The percentage of tumor shrinkage calculated by blended PET-CT, PET-PET and CT-CT registrations using both BSD and FFD are also shown in Table 2 for each case. Quantitatively, using BSD, both PET-PET and CT-CT registrations showed inferior results compared to blended PET-CT. For smaller shrinkage, FFD had similar accuracy to BSD, but its accuracy worsened for larger changes. However using FFD, PET-PET had the worst results while CT-CT achieved much better accuracy. These results aligned with the literature that diffeomorphic algorithm performs better on larger deformations whereas smaller soft tissue changes in CT can be better captured using the FFD algorithm [1].

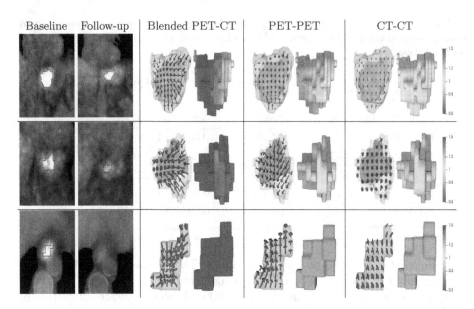

Fig. 3. First column shows baseline and follow-up blended PET-CT images for three tumors in coronal (top, middle) and axial (bottom) views. Red contour is MTV. In the second to the last column, DVF (left) illustrate the change from baseline MTV (green) to follow-up MTV (blue) and Jacobian maps (right) are overlaid on baseline MTV. Color bar indicates shrinkage (blue) to expansion (red) in Jacobian map. (Color figure online)

Table 2. Tumor shrinkage quantified by blended PET-CT, PET-PET and CT-CT registrations compared with ground truth segmentation for each case in Fig. 3.

Registration	Cases	Segmentation	PET-CT	PET-PET	CT-CT
BSD	Top	51%	35%	17%	17%
	Middle	78.5%	58.5%	16%	14%
	Bottom	100%	74.5%	19%	14%
FFD	Top	51%	35%	5.8%	14%
	Middle	78.5%	20%	2.3%	43%
	Bottom	100%	35%	6%	37%

Jacobian maps in Fig. 3 illustrate local non-uniform tumor changes. Quantifying change in a non-residual tumor (Fig. 3 bottom) using DIR is challenging due to a large non-correspondence deformation between the two images. Here, we showed that using blended PET-CT image registration we could generate a DVF to quite accurately measure tumor change owing to the dominant metabolic tumor structures in the baseline image and anatomical structures in the follow-up image that guided the registration.

3.3   Pathologic Tumor Response Prediction

Table 3 lists the p-value and AUC for all predictive Jacobian features compared with clinical features as well as a recent esophageal cancer radiomics study using univariate analysis. Standard Deviation (SD) of Correlation, a texture feature in Jacobian map of tumors using blended PET-CT BSD registration achieved higher AUC = 0.85 compared to PET radiomic features analysis performed by Yip *et al.* [13]. Clinical features in our study were not predictive and none FFD based Jacobian features were significant in differentiating pathologic response.

Table 3. Important Jacobian and clinical features in univariate analysis.

Study	Features	AUC	*p-value*
Yip *et al.* [13]	Run length matrix	0.71–0.81	p < 0.02
Current study	ΔMTV	0.62	0.33
	ΔSUV$_{max}$	0.53	0.81
Blended PET-CT	SD Correlation	0.85	0.006
	SD Energy	0.80	0.01
	Mean Cluster Shade	0.77	0.03
PET-PET	Mean Haralick Correlation	0.81	0.01
	Mean Entropy	0.80	0.02
	Mean Energy	0.75	0.04
CT-CT	SD Long Run High Grey Level	0.79	0.02
	SD Long Run	0.76	0.04
	SD High Grey Level	0.76	0.04

In multivariate analysis, the RF-LASSO model achieved the highest accuracy with only one texture feature - Mean of Cluster Shade extracted from blended PET-CT BSD Jacobian map (Sensitivity = 80.6%, Specificity = 82.6%, Accuracy = 82.3%, AUC = 0.81). However, the performance was worsened when adding more features (Fig. 4(a)). This feature quantified the heterogeneity of the tumor change and responders showed higher values meaning more heterogeneous local MTV changes. Figure 4(b) is the ROC curve of the best model and Fig. 4(c) shows this feature can differentiate response very well. Mean of Cluster Shade was selected as the first feature by LASSO, however SD correlation with the highest AUC in univariate analysis was selected as the third feature in the multivariate model. This may be because LASSO selects the least correlated features and Mean of Cluster Shade had the smallest mean absolute correlation (r = 0.22) among the important distinctive features compared to SD correlation (r = 0.46).

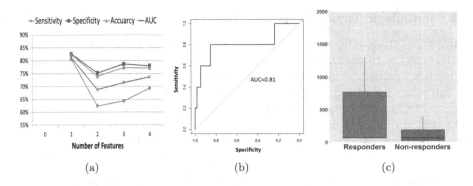

Fig. 4. (a) Model performance with increasing number of features (b) ROC curve on the best model (c) Box plot of Mean of Cluster Shade Jacobian feature.

4 Conclusion and Future Work

We combined PET and CT images into a grayscale blended PET-CT image for quantification of local metabolic tumor change using Jacobian map. We extracted intensity and texture features from the Jacobian map to predict pathologic tumor response in esophageal cancer patients. Jacobian texture features showed the highest accuracy for prediction of pathologic tumor response (accuracy = 82.3%). In the future, we will explore automated optimal weight tuning for PET-CT blending.

References

1. Ashburner, J.: A fast diffeomorphic image registration algorithm. NeuroImage **38**(1), 95–113 (2007)
2. Choi, W., et al.: Radiomics analysis of pulmonary nodules in low-dose CT for early detection of lung cancer. Med. Phys. **45**(4), 1537–1549 (2018)
3. Fuentes, D., et al.: Morphometry-based measurements of the structural response to whole-brain radiation. Int. J. Comput. Assist. Radiol. Surg. **10**(4), 393–401 (2015)
4. Jin, S., Li, D., Wang, H., Yin, Y.: Registration of PET and CT images based on multiresolution gradient of mutual information demons algorithm for positioning esophageal cancer patients. J. Appl. Clin. Med. Phys. **14**(1), 50–61 (2013)
5. Klein, S., Staring, M., Murphy, K., Viergever, M.A., Pluim, J.P.: Elastix: a toolbox for intensity-based medical image registration. IEEE Trans. Med. Imaging **29**(1), 196–205 (2010)
6. Krebs, J., et al.: Robust non-rigid registration through agent-based action learning. In: Descoteaux, M., Maier-Hein, L., Franz, A., Jannin, P., Collins, D.L., Duchesne, S. (eds.) MICCAI 2017. LNCS, vol. 10433, pp. 344–352. Springer, Cham (2017). https://doi.org/10.1007/978-3-319-66182-7_40
7. Staring, M., Klein, S., Pluim, J.P.: A rigidity penalty term for nonrigid registration. Med. Phys. **34**(11), 4098–4108 (2007)
8. Riyahi, S.: Quantifying local tumor morphological changes with Jacobian map for prediction of pathologic tumor response to chemo-radiotherapy in locally advanced esophageal cancer. Phys. Med. Biol. **63**(14), 145020 (2018)

9. Tan, S., Li, L., Choi, W., Kang, M.K., D'Souza, D., Lu, W.: Adaptive region-growing with maximum curvature strategy for tumor segmentation in 18F-FDG PET. Phys. Med. Biol. **62**(13), 5383 (2017)
10. Tustison, N., Avants, B.: Explicit B-spline regularization in diffeomorphic image registration. Front. Neuroinformatics **7**(39), 1–13 (2013)
11. van Velden, F.H.P., Nissen, I.A., Hayes, W., Velasquez, L.M., Hoekstra, O.S., et al.: Effects of reusing baseline volumes of interest by applying (non-)rigid image registration on positron emission tomography response assessments. PloS one **9**(1), e87167 (2014)
12. Westerterp, M., et al.: Esophageal cancer: CT, endoscopic US, and FDG PET for assessment of response to neoadjuvant therapy-systematic review. Radiology **236**(3), 841–851 (2005)
13. Yip, S.S.F., et al.: Relationship between the temporal changes in positron-emission-tomography-imaging-based textural features and pathologic response and survival in esophageal cancer patients. Front. Oncol. **6**, 72 (2016)

Optimizing External Surface Sensor Locations for Respiratory Tumor Motion Prediction

Yusuf Özbek[✉], Zoltan Bardosi, Srdjan Milosavljevic,
and Wolfgang Freysinger

4D Visualization Research Group, Univ. ENT Clinic,
Medical University of Innsbruck, Anichstr. 35, 6020 Innsbruck, Austria
Yusuf.Oezbek@Student.i-med.ac.at

Abstract. Real-time tracking of tumor motion due to the patient's respiratory cycle is a crucial task in radiotherapy treatments. In this work a proof-of-concept setup is presented where real-time tracked external skin attached sensors are used to predict the internal tumor locations. The spatiotemporal relationships between external sensors and targets during the respiratory cycle are modeled using Gaussian Process regression and trained on a preoperative 4D-CT image sequence of the respiratory cycle. A large set ($N \approx 25$) of computer-tomography markers are attached on the patient's skin before CT acquisition to serve as candidate sensor locations from which a smaller subset ($N \approx 6$) is selected based on their combined predictive power using a genetic algorithm based optimization technique. A custom 3D printed sensor-holder design is used to allow accurate positioning of optical or electromagnetic sensors at the best predictive CT marker locations preoperatively, which are then used for real-time prediction of the internal tumor locations. The method is validated on an artificial respiratory phantom model. The model represents the candidate external locations (fiducials) and internal targets (tumors) with CT markers. A 4D-CT image sequence with 11 time-steps at different phases of the respiratory cycles was acquired. Within this test setup, the CT markers for both internal and external structures are automatically determined by a morphology-based algorithm in the CT images. The method's in-sample cross validation accuracy in the training set as given by the average root mean-squared error (RMSE) is between 0.00024 and 0.072 mm.

Keywords: Tumor tracking · Respiratory motion · Prediction
Optimization

1 Problem

The localization of the internal tumors or structures and the detection of respiratory organ or tumor movement under certain therapies (e.g. in radiation

© Springer Nature Switzerland AG 2018
A. Melbourne and R. Licandro et al. (Eds.): DATRA/PIPPI 2018, LNCS 11076, pp. 42–51, 2018.
https://doi.org/10.1007/978-3-030-00807-9_5

therapy or radiofrequency ablation) and real-time visualization of these movements are an important concern in the safe and effective provision of precision radiotherapy, computer-assisted tumor surgery and biopsy. The information on the movements and tracking of the current positions of targeted tumors, e.g. in prostate, liver, lung or soft tissue tumors are traditionally performed by using abdominal compression, breath hold, respiratory gating, implanted radiation-impermeable markers and real-time motion tracking of these markers with optical (OP) or electromagnetic (EM) tracker [1, 2] or over real-time image processing of interventional 4D-CT, -MRI, and 3D/4D-ultrasound [3, 4]. Because of the difficulties with respect to the intraoperative complexity of these methods, there is currently no clinically established solution for the reliable determination of respiratory movements of internal organs, tumors or soft tissues.

Specifically, in the real-time motion tracking of external sensors with OP or EM tracking systems, it is difficult to determine the optimal amount and location of sensors preoperatively that provides sufficient predictions of the internal tumor locations. The used surface markers are randomly distributed [5] and placed on the patient in the near region of a surgical area and all of them are used for respiratory motion prediction, which can increase the error rate in the real-time prediction [6].

2   Materials and Methods

2.1   Phantom Respiratory System Model

The training and evaluation of internal target motion prediction is performed with a custom built phantom model (see Fig. 1). It simulates the most important aspects (with respect to motion prediction) of the human respiratory cycle. The main components consist of a standard rubber hot-water bottle (modeling the abdomen), an internally located spherical rubber balloon (modeling a moving organ). A flexible silicone tube and a water blaster was used to control the amount of air within the model. Sensor-holders within CT skin markers (external input) and skin markers or retro-reflective balls (internal target) are to use in prediction.

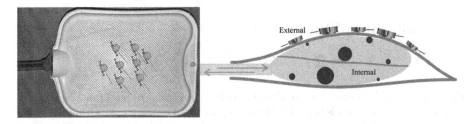

Fig. 1. Left: Respiratory model with the fixed sensor-holders on it. Right: Interior view of the model during an inhalation. The inside of the balloon (max. inflation ⌀ 120 cm) is brought out and a rubber band from both ends of the balloon is glued, so that it stays in the middle, if the outside brought in and inflated. To simulate tumor motion; the X-Spot skin markers (⌀ 1.5 mm) and retro-reflective markers (⌀ 12 mm) are placed inside of the balloon. A flexible silicone tube (L 200 cm, ⌀ 20 mm) is used for inflating the balloon (inhalation/exhalation) with the water blaster (82 × 5 × 15 cm).

2.2   Sensor Holders

The external surface sensors are used in several real-time tumor movement prediction methods [7–11]. In most cases - however - the external sensors are fixed at arbitrary locations that may be sub-optimal for prediction accuracy. Optimizing the spatial distribution and quantity of those surface markers with respect to their prediction power in the preoperative phase therefore can improve the tracking accuracy in the intraoperative phase.

As the two phases typically require different types of external markers, custom made 3D printed sensor-holders were developed (see Fig. 2) to enable switching the sensors while maintaining the same sensor origin. This enables an offline prediction preoperatively using CT markers, and using the pre-trained predictors with a real-time tracking system during the intervention after the known relative transformation between the X-Spot marker and the inserted real-time tracker sensor is applied.

The main part of the sensor-holder consists of an X-Spot CT marker centered in a sensor attachment point. During the preoperative phase, 10–25 of these empty sensor-holders are fixed to the phantom patient. During the intraoperative phase, the sensor-holder can optionally hold an optical- or magnetic-tracking sensor. When used with optical tracking, the sensor-holder can hold an active IRED tracker sensor ($11 \times 7 \times 5$ mm, NDI Optotrak Certus) (Fig. 2(d)). When used with magnetic (EM) tracking, it can hold a 5-DOF NDI Aurora sensor (Length: 8 mm, $\oslash$ 0.6 mm) (Fig. 2(e)) concentrically.

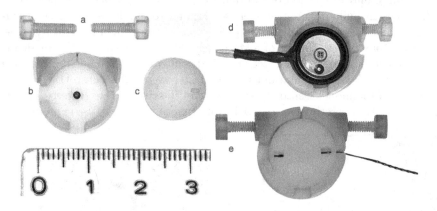

Fig. 2. (a) Two M2 screws that are placed from both directions to establish a rigid setup once an OP or EM sensor is placed in the main part. (b) The main part within a X-Spot marker. It used in offline prediction step. (c) The EM-Sensor-Holder to fix the EM sensor in it. (d) View of sensor-holder within an OP marker. (e) View of sensor-holder within an EM sensor. The parts a, c, d and e are intended for the real-time prediction.

2.3   Data Acquisition

In order to validate sensor optimization, a 4D-CT scan of phantom patient is acquired. The phantom model with 27 external (candidate locations) and 5 internal (target locations) markers in the balloon is placed into the CT device. During the imaging the respiration cycle is simulated by manually adjusting different air amount within the balloon using the water blaster connected to the model with a flexible tube. For the 4D-CT a scanner in Univ. Clinic for Radiology (Siemens healthcare Austria) in Medical Univ. of Innsbruck is used. The scan consists of 11 discrete time steps of a breathing cycle (see Fig. 3). Each axial CT slice (512 × 512 px) has a thickness of 1.0 mm and the 11 discrete CT phases consist of 261 images with 0.488 × 0.488 × 0.488 mm pixel spacing.

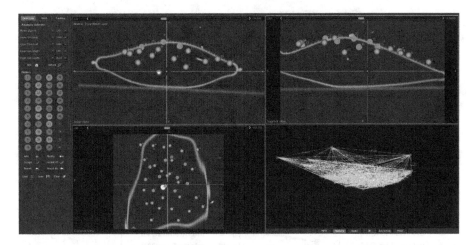

Fig. 3. Detected external markers in the first phase of the visualized 4D-CT images. Left frame is used to set parameters for the automatic marker detection algorithm and contains a marker list for the marker management. The detected markers are inserted into the marker list and visualized in the standard DICOM views (axial, sagittal, coronal) in the tiled right window. The green blobs are accepted automatically as external markers (based on given geometrical properties in the detection algorithm) and blue blobs are possible candidates to be accepted manually. The geometry view (right bottom) represents the distances of all detected markers. (Color figure online)

2.4   Automatic Marker Detection

In order to learn the respiratory cycle of the patient from the observed CT images, where the optimal sensor locations for prediction are determined, a regressor is trained to predict internal motion given this data. The precise locations of external and internal fiducials in the CT image space are detected by a GPU accelerated volumetric detection method [12].

For this purpose, each of 11 CT phases are thresholded and binarized to determine the centroid of the fiducials. On the resulting image the 3D fiducials are filtered for spherical structures using morphological opening with a spherical struc-
turing ball element of the appropriate scale given the voxel size of the dataset and
the physical dimensions of the markers. Using a geometry filter on the resulting
spherical blobs best candidates are selected based on shape and size. From the
best candidates the blob centroids are calculated and stored to be used in the prediction step (see Fig. 4).

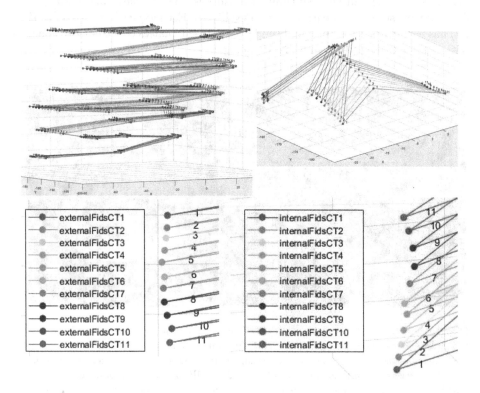

Fig. 4. Top Left: Discrete chronological 3D movement positions of all external surface
fiducials during in-/exhalation over 11 timesteps (Timestep 1: Fully inhaled, Timestep
11: Fully exhaled). The location coordinates are obtained by automatic marker detection. Bottom left: The positions of one external fiducial in 4D-CT image space. Movement positions of internal fiducials in top right and bottom right.

2.5   Determining Surface Sensor Locations with GA

In order to train an accurate prediction of tumor motion from a few optimally positioned fiducials, a multi-objective genetic algorithm (GA) based feature selection
method (similar to [13, 14]) is proposed.

Before the imaging step, a larger set of CT markers $\{c_k\}$, $k \approx 25$ are fixed on the surface at randomized candidate locations.

After imaging, all external surface marker locations are detected. This results in k time-series, each with T timesteps and 3 output dimensions (the spatial coordinates of the sensor in the CT reference frame). The target marker locations over the T timesteps yield the time-series $y \in R^{T \times 3}$.

An individual during the GA search is represented by an element of a k-dimensional binary vector $I = \{0,1\}^k$, where the nth bit represents whether the nth external sensor is used for prediction (1) or not (0).

If a marker is used, its x, y, z coordinates within the CT reference frame are added to the input coordinate set used for prediction. This yields a $3 \times p$ dimensional input feature for each time-step, where p is the number of enabled markers within the individual.

For each individual I, the fitness function is defined by a multi-objective function $F(I) = (F_1(I), S(I))$.

The primary component is given by the weighted sum

$$F_1(I) = E(I) + \alpha * \min(0, S(I) - K)$$

where $E(I)$ is the average RMS error between the predicted and target locations using X as the input feature set over a 3-fold cross-validation on the T timesteps and $S(I)$ is the number of features enabled, K is the maximum preferred number of enabled fiducials and α is a scaling parameter, which balances the trade-off between additional prediction error and the number of enabled fiducials. This setup leads to an optimization goal of finding the minimum achievable prediction error with as few sensors as possible, but softly punishing configurations that have more than K enabled sensors.

For each individual, the predictions are evaluated using 3 Gaussian Process Regressors (GPR) $(G_i : X \rightarrow t_i, i = 1, 2, 3)$ for each coordinate of the target, with C*SE + W where C is constant kernel, SE is squared exponential and W is white noise kernel [15]. (see Fig. 5).

The C kernel is configured with the constant value: 1.0, constant value bounds: 1e−3, 1e3, SE with length scale: 10.0, length scale bounds: 1e−2, 1e2 and W with noise level: 0.1 and noise level bounds: 1e−10, 1e+0.5. The Gaussian Process Regressor is configured with normalized target value without an optimizer. In GA, the parameters for population: 600, cv-proba: 0.5, mu-proba: 0.2, generation: 50, cv-independent-proba: 0.5 and mu-independent-proba: 0.05 are used.

3   Results

Table 1 represents the prediction results for 5 internal target markers in the balloon using automatically recommended surface marker list. Each input marker in the recommended surface sensor group is processed with the listed individual target respectively. The best result is obtained from the C*SE + W of the GPR algorithm. The prediction is performed with a raw data for each surface and target marker respectively.

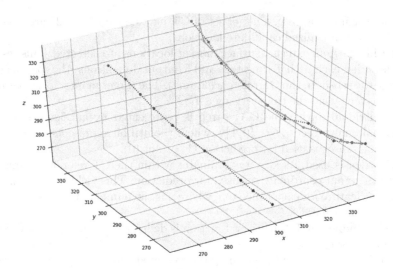

Fig. 5. Prediction result (green dotted lines) for target 1 (red) based on surface marker 8 (blue) from the recommended group (8 and 14) in 11 different time-steps. (Color figure online)

Table 1. Overview of the offline prediction results. The RMS is the average mean squared error of the deviations in each timestep when using the recommended surface sensors.

Internal target	Optimal amount of Surface sensors	Recommended surface sensors	Used Kernel	Used data	Mean prediction RMS
1	2	(8 and 14)	C*SE+W	11 × 3	0.00024
2	6	(1, 3, 7, 12, 18 and 25)			0.0014
3	9	(5, 6, 7, 8, 13, 19, 25, 26 and 27)			0.0023
4	1	(22)			0.072
5	4	(2, 3, 8 and 25)			0.014

4   Discussion

In many treatments, where respiratory motion prediction and tracking is a necessary approach to apply, the success of a treatment strongly depends on the accuracy of prediction, which is related to the detection and placement of the external surface marker locations on the patient.

Therefore, the quantity, location and distribution of the sensors is important and challenging during real-time tumor motion prediction. In the most clinical approaches, the location of external markers is chosen empirically; that is, operator-dependent [5]. Within this work, we examined that the distribution and selection of the best placement locations automatically and intelligently, which gives better prediction results with using less numbers of external sensors to use e.g. in the thorax or abdominal regions. The proposed method is tested through a custom built respiratory phantom model to provide the required dataset, that surrogates same breathing circle of a real patient [16] (Table 2).

Table 2. The 3D positional movement variations of the internal target markers (marker centroids) from fully exhaled to fully inhaled time-steps after 4D-CT.

Internal target marker	1	2	3	4	5
3D Movements in mm x y z	0.69	6.52	6.21	−4.05	1.8
	6.44	17.6	16.57	3.1	1.97
	1.51	2.39	1.4	−9.47	6.58

The primary aim of this work was to separate the preoperative and intraoperative phase based on offline prediction method using sensor-holders. (see Fig. 6). Having already optimal sensor amount and locations with the GPR and GA before intervention also optimizes the whole complex workflow of the real-time respiratory motion prediction and serves a reliable solution to this complexity. All processes in intraoperative phase workflow will be evaluated in the future on the phantom model and real patients to validate the presented approach. The OP or EM tracker will serve sensor data to be used as input for the real-time GPR.

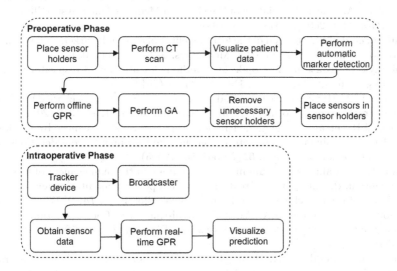

Fig. 6. Current (preoperative phase) and future (intraoperative phase) workflow of the presented work.

5 Conclusion

In this work, a method is presented to automatically determine the optimal locations of the external OP/EM sensors on the patient's surface to predict internal tumor motions with high accuracy. The preoperatively determined optimal sensor locations can be used in real-time tumor motion tracking using the sensors of NDI Optotrak Certus or NDI Aurora tracking systems.

The experiments and evaluations on the built realistic respiratory phantom model have shown that by using our method, best possible locations of surface sensors can be determined with high accuracy and serves a reliable prediction, based on the selected tumor inside the phantom. The experiments give also information the distributing of recommended sensors locations have a high correlation between the surface motion and the internal tumor motion. With this procedure, EM or OP 3D measurement technologies can be used for real-time prediction and it is suitable for use in the medical environment.

References

1. Balter, J.M., et al.: Accuracy of a wireless localization system for radiotherapy. Int. J. Radiat. Oncol. Biol. Phys. **61**(3), 933–7 (2005)
2. Krilavicius, T., Zliobaite, I., Simonavicius, H., Jaruevicius, L.: Predicting respiratory motion for real-time tumour tracking in radiotherapy. In: IEEE 29th International Symposium on Computer-Based Medical Systems (CBMS), June 2016. ISSN: 2372-9198
3. Lee, S.J., Motai, Y.: Prediction and Classification of Respiratory Motion. Springer, Heidelberg (2014). ISBN: 978-3-642-41508-1
4. AAPM Task Group 76: The Management of Respiratory Motion in Radiation Oncology, American Association of Physicists in Medicine One Physics Ellipse, College Park, MD (2006). ISBN: 1-888340-61-4
5. Yan, H., et al.: Investigation of the location effect of external markers in respiratory-gated radiotherapy. J. Appl. Clin. Med. Phys. **9**(2), 57–68 (2008)
6. Spinczyk, D., Karwan, A., Copik, M.: Methods for abdominal respiratory motion tracking. Comput. Aided Surg. **19**(1–3), 34–47 (2014)
7. Buzurovic, I., Huang, K., Yu, Y., Podder, T.K.: A robotic approach to 4D real-time tumor tracking for radiotherapy. Phys. Med. Biol. **56**(5), 1299–1318 (2011)
8. Wong, J.R., et al.: Image-guided radiotherapy for prostate cancer by CT-linear accelerator combination: prostate movements and dosimetric considerations. Int. J. Radiat. Oncol. Biol. Phys. **61**(2), 561–569 (2005)
9. Sawant, A., et al.: Toward submillimeter accuracy in the management of intrafraction motion: the integration of real-time internal position monitoring and multileaf collimator target tracking. Int. J. Radiat. Oncol. Biol. Phys. **74**(2), 575–582 (2009)
10. D'Souza, W.D., Naqvi, S.A., Yu, C.X.: Real-time intra-fraction-motion tracking using the treatment couch: a feasibility study. Phys. Med. Biol. **50**(17), 4021–4033 (2005)
11. Buzurovic, I., Podder, T.K., Huang, K., Yu, Y.: Tumor motion prediction and tracking in adaptive radiotherapy. In: IEEE International Conference on Bioinformatics and Bioengineering, pp. 273–278 (2010)

12. Bardosi, Z.: OpenCL accelerated GPU binary morphology image filters for ITK. Insight Journal (2015)
13. Spolaôr, N., Lorena, A.C., Lee, H.D.: Multi-objective genetic algorithm evaluation in feature selection. In: Takahashi, R.H.C., Deb, K., Wanner, E.F., Greco, S. (eds.) EMO 2011. LNCS, vol. 6576, pp. 462–476. Springer, Heidelberg (2011). https://doi.org/10.1007/978-3-642-19893-9_32
14. Goldberg, D.E.: Genetic Algorithms in Search, Optimization, and Machine Learning, 1st edn. Addison-Wesley Professional (1989). ISBN: 978-0201157673
15. Rasmussen, C., Williams, C.: Gaussian Processes for Machine Learning. MIT University Press Group Ltd. (2005). ISBN: 026218253X
16. Weiss, E., Wijesooriya, K., Dill, S.V., Keall, P.J.: Tumor and normal tissue motion in the thorax during respiration analysis of volumetric and positional variations using 4D CT. Int. J. Radiation Oncol. Biol. Phys. **67**(1), 296–307 (2007)

PIPPI

प्रभाग

Segmentation of Fetal Adipose Tissue Using Efficient CNNs for Portable Ultrasound

Sagar Vaze and Ana I. L. Namburete[✉]

Institute of Biomedical Engineering, Department of Engineering Science,
University of Oxford, Oxford, UK
`ana.namburete@eng.ox.ac.uk`

Abstract. Adipose tissue mass has been shown to have a strong correlation with fetal nourishment, which has consequences on health in infancy and later life. In rural areas of developing nations, ultrasound has the potential to be the key imaging modality due to its portability and cost. However, many ultrasound image analysis algorithms are not compatibly portable, with many taking several minutes to compute on modern CPUs.

The contributions of this work are threefold. Firstly, by adapting the popular U-Net, we show that CNNs can achieve excellent results in fetal adipose segmentation from ultrasound images. We then propose a reduced model, `U-Ception`, facilitating deployment of the algorithm on mobile devices. The `U-Ception` network provides a 98.4% reduction in model size for a 0.6% reduction in segmentation accuracy (mean Dice coefficient). We also demonstrate the clinical applicability of the work, showing that CNNs can be used to predict a trend between gestational age and adipose area.

1 Introduction

Ultrasound has the potential to be the key imaging modality in rural areas of developing nations, due to its low cost and portability. To complement this portability, there is a need for image analysis tools which are similarly mobile, allowing them to be implemented alongside the imaging itself in remote locations. The most practical mode of deployment would be an application on an iOS or Android device, such as a tablet or mobile phone, which typically come with hardware limitations such as smaller RAM and less powerful GPUs.

However, current ultrasound analysis techniques are not compatibly efficient, with many taking several minutes to run on modern CPUs [1]. Furthermore, most convolutional neural networks (CNNs) - which are currently state-of-the-art in image analysis tasks - require too much memory to deploy on a mobile phone or tablet. In response to this, we propose a novel CNN architecture, `U-Ception`, which uses *depth-wise separable convolutions* to analyze ultrasound images in a computationally efficient manner.

A. Melbourne and R. Licandro et al. (Eds.): DATRA/PIPPI 2018, LNCS 11076, pp. 55–65, 2018.
https://doi.org/10.1007/978-3-030-00807-9_6

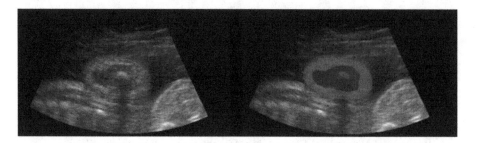

Fig. 1. Cross-sectional image of fetal a arm (left), with segmentation (right). Segmentation shows adipose tissue (of interest, blue), muscle (red), and humerus (green). (Color figure online)

The target application is the segmentation of fetal adipose tissue, as shown in Fig. 1. It has been shown that adipose mass has a 'pronounced sensitivity' to maternal - and thus fetal - nutritional state [2]. This is of special importance in the developing world, where 152 of the world's 155 million stunted under-five year olds reside [3]. Thus, the observation and control of fetal nourishment is crucial: developmentally, the most important time for proper nourishment is in the first 1000 days (from conception until the 2nd birthday), and catch-up growth in later childhood is 'minimal' [4].

This work presents the U-Ception network: a CNN designed for segmentation of adipose tissue in fetal ultrasound data. Firstly, in Sect. 2, this work summarizes previous efforts at fetal segmentation, and a number of popular methods which reduce neural network size. Section 3 will then describe the CNNs proposed for this segmentation challenge. The first - an adaptation of the popular 'U-Net' [5] - provides a baseline performance against which the reduced U-Ception architecture can be compared. Section 4 describes the experimental set-up, and Sect. 5 outlines our results, showing the similarity in performance between the adapted U-Net and U-Ception models.

2   Previous Work

The current state-of-the-art in fetal adipose segmentation is the feature asymmetry approach proposed by Rueda et al. [6]. Feature asymmetry is a phase-based method, which uses points of phase congruency at specific frequencies to build an edge map which is robust to changes in contrast. Other approaches to fetal ultrasound segmentation include the use of active contours [7,8], Hough transforms [9] and multi-level thresholding [1].

However, for most biomedical image segmentation, the most prevalent algorithms are convolutional neural networks (CNNs). An important CNN is the 'U-Net' [5], which has been used extensively in the biomedical field [10,11]. The network won the ISBI neuronal segmentation challenge in 2015 by a significant margin - despite a small training set of 30 images - by performing strong data augmentation. It is adapted in this work: first to form a baseline for the application of CNNs to fetal adipose segmentation, and then as a guide for the proposed CNN with a smaller 'size'.

Network size is defined as its memory footprint, which is directly proportional to the number of its parameters, and is the main bottleneck in the application of CNNs on mobile devices. Mobile devices typically come with between 2 GB and 4 GB of RAM, with many modern networks (especially segmentation architectures) having hundreds of millions of parameters, with sizes nearing a gigabyte.

Numerous efforts have been made to reduce neural network size by efficiently storing these parameters. Wu et al. quantized the weights of the network, learning an optimal quantization codebook using K-Means clustering [12]. Huffman coding (a lossless method of compressing data) has also been used to efficiently store network weights [13].

Another method of building a smaller network is distillation [14]. Distillation is the process of using a larger network to train a smaller network, passing on the generalization ability of the large network.

A class of techniques seeks to factorize the convolutions in the networks, breaking them down into a number of steps. One example of this was suggested by Jin et al., which, instead of convolving feature maps with 3D tensors, decomposes the process into convolutions with three one-dimensional vectors [15].

This work uses *depth-wise separable convolutions* [16], which have been shown to provide high accuracy results in the 'Xception' classification network [17]. The latest model from Google DeepLab ('DeepLab v3+' [18]) adapts the Xception network for segmentation purposes. Depth-wise separable convolutions were chosen for this work as they factorize the 3D convolution in an intuitive fashion, breaking the process into spatial and channel-wise components (see Sect. 3.2).

3 Architecture Design

3.1 Adapted U-Net

The 'U-Net' [5] was first adapted to provide a baseline performance for neural networks in the context of fetal adipose segmentation. The encoder path of the network contains two convolutional layers (13×13 kernels, see Sect. 4) followed by max-pooling, repeated 4 times, resulting in a reduction of spatial channel dimensions by a factor of 16. With each down-sampling layer the number of feature channels is doubled, with 48 channels in the first layer, and 768 channels in the lowest. The decoder is symmetrical, but with up-sampling in place of max-pooling. The final layer is a 1×1 convolutional layer.

All convolutional layers were zero-padded, with all but the final layer using the ReLU non-linearity. The final layer uses a sigmoidal activation to map network predictions to values between 0 and 1, with scores close to 1 indicating a confident prediction of adipose tissue at a pixel location.

3.2   Reduced U-Net: U-Ception

This section describes the efforts made to reduce the number of parameters in the segmentation network, and hence the size of the model's parameter file. The proposed method uses *depth-wise separable convolutions*, which were used successfully in the 'Xception' network [17]. These convolutions were applied to the U-Net architecture, with the resulting architecture termed U-Ception.

The proposed architecture is essentially identical to the adapted U-Net, but with more feature channels per layer, and all convolutional layers replaced with separable convolutional layers. This modification leads to a drastic reduction in the network's parameter count, from **296 million** to **4.6 million** parameters. The architecture is detailed in Fig. 2.

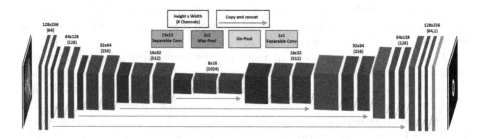

Fig. 2. U-Ception architecture

Depth-Wise Separable Convolutions: Regular convolutional layers in CNNs involve convolutions with three-dimensional kernels. Two of these dimensions are spatial, and are responsible for combining data from a single channel, in a similar manner to convolution filters in classical image processing. The third dimension, however, is responsible for combining information from all of the feature channels, such that new feature maps can be produced. The number of parameters in the convolution tensor for a layer, therefore, can be described by Eq. 1. Here, K is the spatial dimension of the square filter, N is the number of input channels, and M the number of output channels. Note that K^2N parameters are required to compute each of the M output feature maps. The process is illustrated in Fig. 3(a).

$$n_{parameters} = K^2NM \qquad K, N, M \in \mathbb{Z}^+ \tag{1}$$

The idea behind depth-wise separable convolutions is to separate the convolutions in the spatial dimensions and the channel dimension. First, one feature map is calculated per input channel by spatially convolving each input channel with a single filter. Next, the output is fed to a regular convolutional layer with $1 \times 1 \times N$ kernel size, so the information across input channels can be combined. In this way, the multiplicative interaction between the N input channels and M

output channels is not scaled by the squared spatial kernel size, K^2. The number of parameters in this new layer is described by Eq. 2.

$$n_{parameters} = K^2N + \bar{K}^2NM = K^2N + NM \qquad K, N, M \in \mathbb{Z}^+ \qquad (2)$$

Note that the variable $\bar{K} = 1$ is introduced to illustrate that the second stage of convolutions is identical to a regular convolutional layer with a spatial kernel size of 1. Also, in some implementations, a channel multiplier C_m is introduced such that, in the spatial convolution stage, C_m intermediate feature maps are produced per input channel. This would scale the number of parameters in the depth-wise separable layer by C_m. In this work, a channel multiplier of 1 is used. The process is shown in Fig. 3(b).

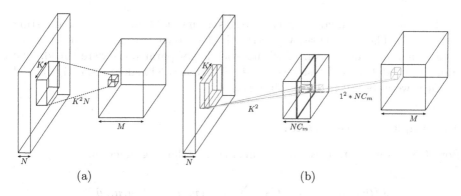

(a)   (b)

Fig. 3. (a) Regular convolutional layer. Here convolution occurs with a tensor with square spatial dimensions K, and depth equal to the number of input channels, N. Each of the M filters requires K^2N parameters. (b) Separable convolutional layer. Here each input feature channel is convolved separately with C_m tensors with depth of 1 and spatial dimensions of K. The resulting feature maps are convolved with M tensors of depth NC_m and spatial dimensions of 1. In this work, layers with $C_m = 1$ are used.

4   Experimental Setup

4.1   Fetal Dataset

Data for this task was collected as part of the INTERGROWTH-21st Project, with 324 3D ultrasound volumes of healthy fetal arms acquired. From each volume, five 2D slices were extracted perpendicular to the humerus and annotated by one of three experts, delineating the adipose tissue, as shown in Fig. 4. The images were collected with a Philips HD9 ultrasound machine (resolution of 0.99 mm per voxel), with the subjects' gestational ages ranging from 17 to 41 weeks. The dataset is a larger sample of that used by Rueda et al. [6] (the previous effort at fetal adipose segmentation).

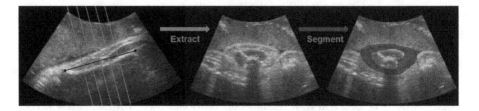

Fig. 4. Extraction and segmentation of 2D slices from an ultrasound volume. Left-most image shows a sagittal view of the fetal humerus. Red points show humerus end points and yellow lines indicate slice planes. Intersections of the red and yellow lines - the yellow points - show centers of extracted slices. Also shown is one extracted slice (middle) and its segmentation (right). (Color figure online)

The dataset was divided with an 80–20 split into folds for training and testing respectively. The training set was further broken down, with 20% of the 2D slices used as a validation set, on which network hyper-parameters were tuned. The training, validation and test sets had 1100, 270 and 340 slices respectively, and all slices were resized to 128×256 pixels.

4.2   Implementation Details

Both CNNs were optimized by maximizing the following function:

$$\mathcal{L}(\boldsymbol{\theta}; \boldsymbol{y}, \hat{\boldsymbol{y}}) = -\lambda_1 ||\boldsymbol{\theta}||_2 + \sum_{i=1}^{n} IoU(\boldsymbol{y_i}, \hat{\boldsymbol{y_i}}) + \lambda_2 h(\boldsymbol{y_i}, \hat{\boldsymbol{y_i}}) \tag{3}$$

Here, $\boldsymbol{y}$ and $\hat{\boldsymbol{y}}$ represent the manual training labels and the network predictions respectively, while $\boldsymbol{\theta}$ represents the CNN parameters. IoU represents the intersection-over-union score of the manual labels and the network predictions, with λ_1 signifying the weight decay strength. The function h represents a boundary regularizer, which explicitly penalizes incorrect network predictions at the adipose boundaries.

Optimization was done with stochastic gradient descent, reducing the learning rate by a factor of 10 every 15 epochs. Both networks were implemented using Keras (TensorFlow backend), with training done on an NVIDIA Quadro P5000 GPU. Interestingly, independent optimization of both the adapted U-Net and the U-Ception models showed that both networks had identical optimal hyper-parameter settings. An initial learning rate of 1×10^{-2} was used, with λ_1 (weight decay) set to 1×10^{-2}, and λ_2 (boundary regularizer strength) to 1×10^{-3}. Furthermore, batch normalization was used on all layer inputs, and dropout regularization was used on the input layer and lowest layer ($p = 0.2$ and $p = 0.5$ respectively) as in the original U-Net. Kernels of size 13×13 were used in both networks to deal with the large areas of adipose discontinuity in the images (a product of ultrasound shadows).

5   Results and Discussion

This section compares the performances of the regular convolution U-Net and U-Ception networks on a held-out test set of 340 slices (extracted from 68 volumes).

Sample qualitative results are shown in Fig. 5. It can be seen that the networks generally capture the adipose tissue well, with both learning to predict closed-ring segmentations, even in the presence of adipose signal occlusion (for instance, the vertical shadow below the humerus). Failure modes are also shown (Dice coefficient < 0.5), with failure occurring in the presence of a sparse signal (Example 6), or when the target slice has many distracting shapes (Example 7).

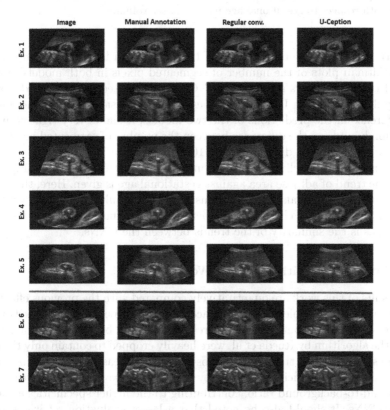

Fig. 5. Sample results from the CNNs on a held-out test set. Failure modes are shown in Examples 6 and 7. Note that a disproportionate number of failure modes are shown.

A chi-square test was performed on the Dice coefficients produced by the U-Net and U-Ception models on the test set. It was found that there is no statistically significant difference between the U-Ception's Dice distribution and that of the regular U-Net ($p \approx 1.00$). Though this p value is high, it is perhaps unsurprising given the visual similarities of the two models' results (see Fig. 5).

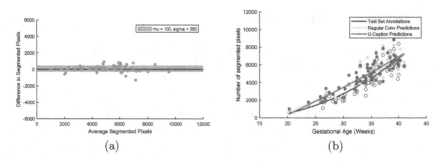

Fig. 6. (a) Bland-Altman plot of the number of segmented pixels in `U-Ception` model against regular convolution model. (b) Adipose area trend (in number of segmented pixels) with respect to gestational age using test set volumes.

Further insight into performance of the models can be gained by inspecting Bland-Altman plots of the number of segmented pixels in both models' predictions. Figure 6(a) shows a plot of the `U-Ception` architecture compared against the regular convolution U-Net. This diagram suggests strongly that there is little difference in the predictions of the two models; it shows very tight standard deviation bounds on the difference between the number of segmented pixels, and a similarly small mean difference ($\mu = 100, \sigma = 380$).

An example of the clinical applications of the algorithms is given in Fig. 6(b), where the trend of adipose area against gestational age is given. Here, the trends computed using the manual annotations and CNN results are given for all volumes in the test set. The similarity between the manual and CNN trends is evident, as is the similarity of the trends between the CNNs.

5.1   Comparison with Previous Work

The results of this work are quantitatively compared with the previous efforts by Rueda et al. [6] in Table 1. Here, the accuracy (sensitivity and specificity) and Dice are detailed. To contextualize the results, it should be noted that the images fed to the algorithm by Rueda et al. were heavily cropped to contain only the area of interest. This makes the task of adipose localization easier, contributing to the higher mean Dice coefficient achieved by the previous work. It also increases the foreground-to-background ratio, contributing to the higher specificities achieved by the CNNs. It should also be noted that a larger evaluation set was used in this work - 340 slices, in contrast to the 81 slices in the work by Rueda et al. - contributing to the larger standard deviations in our results.

Nonetheless, the classical algorithm outperforms the CNNs in terms of Dice coefficient, while the CNNs achieve better results with respect to both accuracy metrics. Also, the `U-Ception` network gives a small but not statistically significant compromise in performance when compared against the regular convolution U-Net.

Table 1. Comparison of method by Rueda et al. [6] against the proposed CNNs ($\mu \pm \sigma$).

	Sensitivity (%)	Specificity (%)	Dice (%)
Rueda et al.	87.30 ± 3.84	97.05 ± 1.17	**87.11 ± 2.60**
Regular conv.	**88.29 ± 12.15**	**98.85 ± 0.75**	80.89 ± 13.75
U-Ception	87.45 ± 13.30	98.71 ± 0.83	80.25 ± 11.50

5.2 Comparing Algorithm Efficiencies

Table 2 summarizes the two model sizes and prediction times of both networks on a CPU and on a variety of portable devices. The CPU prediction times are averaged over 100 samples. The times shown compare favorably with those required for classical techniques - many of which take several minutes to run on a modern CPU [1].

Table 2. Model sizes of both networks, as well as prediction times on a range of hardware. Note that the regular convolution model was too large to deploy on the mobile devices.

	Model size	i5-4200M CPU	Google Pixel 2	Samsung Galaxy S5	Samsung Galaxy Tab A
Regular conv.	1.10 GB	15.8 s	N/A	N/A	N/A
U-Ception	18 MB	2.7 s	≈4 s	≈8 s	≈11 s

The table also shows that, with modern hardware, even the large network can make a prediction in reasonable time (15.8 s), as the number of FLOPs required for a forward pass rises only linearly with the number of parameters in the network. Thus, the main bottleneck in implementation of these networks on a mobile device is clarified: the size of the weight file. Typically, TensorFlow stores each parameter as a 32-bit float, meaning a network with 20 million parameters will have a weight file of approximately 75 MB in size. The regular convolution U-Net has **296 million** parameters, with the resulting weight file taking **1.10 GB** on disk. The U-Ception architecture requires only **4.6 million** parameters, with a weight file of **18 MB**. Thus the model provides a reduction in both weight file size and parameter count of **98.4%**, while achieving similar performance on the test set (with a 0.6% compromise in mean Dice coefficient).

6 Conclusion

This work proposes an end-to-end framework for the semantic segmentation of fetal adipose tissue using convolutional neural networks. Furthermore, a highly efficient novel network architecture - `U-Ception` - is proposed, using depth-wise separable convolutions to reduce model parameter count. It is shown that the `U-Ception` architecture's performance is statistically equivalent to that of the regular convolution U-Net, with the benefit of a 98.4% reduction in model size.

Acknowledgements. The authors are grateful for support from the Royal Academy of Engineering under the Engineering for Development Research Fellowship scheme, and the INTERGROWTH-21st Consortium for provision of 3D fetal US image data.

References

1. Rueda, S., et al.: Evaluation and comparison of current fetal ultrasound image segmentation methods for biometric measurements: a grand challenge. IEEE Trans. Med. Imaging **33**(4), 797–813 (2014)
2. Symonds, M.E., Mostyn, A., Pearce, S., Budge, H., Stephenson, T.: Endocrine and nutritional regulation of fetal adipose tissue development. J. Endocrinol. **179**(3), 293–299 (2003)
3. UNICEF: Joint Malnutrition Estimates 2017 - UNICEF Data and Analytics
4. Lloyd-Fox, S., et al.: Functional near infrared spectroscopy (fNIRS) to assess cognitive function in infants in rural Africa. Nat. Sci. Rep. **4**, 1–8 (2014)
5. Ronneberger, O., Fischer, P., Brox, T.: U-Net: convolutional networks for biomedical image segmentation. In: Navab, N., Hornegger, J., Wells, W.M., Frangi, A.F. (eds.) MICCAI 2015. LNCS, vol. 9351, pp. 234–241. Springer, Cham (2015). https://doi.org/10.1007/978-3-319-24574-4_28
6. Rueda, S., Knight, C.L., Papageorghiou, A.T., Alison Noble, J.: Feature-based fuzzy connectedness segmentation of ultrasound images with an object completion step. Med. Image Anal. **26**(1), 30–46 (2015)
7. Chalana, V., Winter, T.C., Cyr, D.R., Haynor, D.R., Kim, Y.: Automatic fetal head measurements from sonographic images. Acad. Radiol. **3**(8), 628–635 (1996)
8. Pathak, S.D., Chalana, V., Kim, Y.: Interactive automatic fetal head measurements from ultrasound images using multimedia computer technology. Ultrasound Med. Biol. **23**(5), 665–673 (1997)
9. Lu, W., Tan, J., Floyd, R.: Automated fetal head detection and measurement in ultrasound images by iterative randomized hough transform. Ultrasound Med. Biol. **31**(7), 929–936 (2005)
10. Çiçek, Ö., Abdulkadir, A., Lienkamp, S.S., Brox, T., Ronneberger, O.: 3D U-Net: learning dense volumetric segmentation from sparse annotation. In: Ourselin, S., Joskowicz, L., Sabuncu, M.R., Unal, G., Wells, W. (eds.) MICCAI 2016. LNCS, vol. 9901, pp. 424–432. Springer, Cham (2016). https://doi.org/10.1007/978-3-319-46723-8_49
11. Ravishankar, H., Venkataramani, R., Thiruvenkadam, S., Sudhakar, P., Vaidya, V.: Learning and incorporating shape models for semantic segmentation. In: Descoteaux, M., Maier-Hein, L., Franz, A., Jannin, P., Collins, D.L., Duchesne, S. (eds.) MICCAI 2017. LNCS, vol. 10433, pp. 203–211. Springer, Cham (2017). https://doi.org/10.1007/978-3-319-66182-7_24

12. Wu, J., Leng, C., Wang, Y., Hu, Q., Cheng, J.: Quantized convolutional neural networks for mobile devices. In: CVPR (2016)
13. Han, S., Mao, H., Dally, W.J.: Deep compression: compressing deep neural networks with pruning, trained quantization and Huffman coding. In: ICLR (2016)
14. Hinton, G., Vinyals, O., Dean, J.: Distilling the knowledge in a neural network. In: NIPS Deep Learning Workshop (2015)
15. Jin, J., Dundar, A., Culurciello, E.: Flattened convolutional neural networks for feedforward acceleration. In: ICLR (2015)
16. Sifre, L., Mallat, S.: Rigid-motion scattering for image classification. Ecole Polytechnique, CMAP. Ph.D. thesis (2014)
17. Chollet, F.: Xception: deep learning with depthwise separable convolutions. In: CVPR (2016)
18. Chen, W., et al.: Compressing neural networks with the hashing trick. ICML (2015)

Automatic Shadow Detection in 2D Ultrasound Images

Qingjie Meng[1](✉), Christian Baumgartner[2], Matthew Sinclair[1],
James Housden[3], Martin Rajchl[1], Alberto Gomez[3], Benjamin Hou[1],
Nicolas Toussaint[3], Veronika Zimmer[3], Jeremy Tan[1], Jacqueline Matthew[3],
Daniel Rueckert[1], Julia Schnabel[3], and Bernhard Kainz[1]

[1] Biomedical Image Analysis Group, Imperial College London, London, UK
`q.meng16@imperial.ac.uk`
[2] Computer Vision Lab, ETH Zürich, Zürich, Switzerland
[3] School of Biomedical Engineering and Imaging Sciences,
Kings College London, London, UK

Abstract. Automatically detecting acoustic shadows is of great importance for automatic 2D ultrasound analysis ranging from anatomy segmentation to landmark detection. However, variation in shape and similarity in intensity to other structures make shadow detection a very challenging task. In this paper, we propose an automatic shadow detection method to generate a pixel-wise, shadow-focused confidence map from weakly labelled, anatomically-focused images. Our method: (1) initializes potential shadow areas based on a classification task. (2) extends potential shadow areas using a GAN model. (3) adds intensity information to generate the final confidence map using a distance matrix. The proposed method accurately highlights the shadow areas in 2D ultrasound datasets comprising standard view planes as acquired during fetal screening. Moreover, the proposed method outperforms the state-of-the-art quantitatively and improves failure cases for automatic biometric measurement.

1 Introduction

2D Ultrasound (US) imaging is a popular medical imaging modality based on reflection and scattering of high frequency sound in tissue, well known for its portability, low cost, and high temporal resolution. However, this modality is inherently prone to artefacts in clinical practice due to low energies used and the physical nature of sound waves propagation in tissue. Artefacts such as noise, distortions and acoustic shadows are unavoidable, and have a significant impact on the achievable image quality. Noise can be handled through better hardware and advanced image reconstruction algorithms [7], while distortions can be tackled by operator training and knowledge of the underlying anatomy [15]. However, acoustic shadows are more challenging to resolve.

Acoustic shadows are caused by sound-opaque occluders, which can potentially conceal vital anatomical information. Shadow regions have low signal

© Springer Nature Switzerland AG 2018
A. Melbourne and R. Licandro et al. (Eds.): DATRA/PIPPI 2018, LNCS 11076, pp. 66–75, 2018.
https://doi.org/10.1007/978-3-030-00807-9_7

intensity with very high acoustic impedance differences at the boundaries. Sonographers are trained to avoid acoustic shadows by using real-time acquisition devices. Shadows are either avoided by moving to a more preferable viewing direction or, if no shadow-free viewing direction can be found, a mental map is compounded with iterative acquisitions from different orientations. Although acoustic shadows may be useful for practitioners to determine the anatomical properties of occluders, images containing strong shadows can be problematic for automatic real-time image analysis methods which, such as; provide directional guidance; perform biometric measurements; or automatic evaluate biomarkers, etc. Therefore shadow-aware US image analysis would beneficial for many of these applications, as well as clinical practice.

Contribution: (1) We propose a novel method that uses weak annotations (shadow/shadow-free images) to generate an anatomically agnostic shadow confidence map in 2D ultrasound images; (2) The proposed method achieves accurate shadow detection visually and quantitatively for different fetal anatomies; (3) To our knowledge, this is the first shadow detection model for ultrasound images that generates a dense, shadow-focused confidence map; (4) The proposed shadow detection method can be used in real-time automatic US image analysis, such as anatomical segmentation and registration. In our experiments, the obtained shadow confidence map greatly improves segmentation performance of failure cases in automatic biometric measurement.

Related Work: US artefacts have been well studied in clinical literature, e.g. [5,13] provide an overview. However, anatomically agnostic acoustic shadow detection has rarely been the focus within the medical image analysis community. [10] developed a shadow detection method based on geometrical modelling of the US B-Mode cone with statistical tests. This is an anatomical-specific technique designed to detect only a subset of 'deep' acoustic shadows, which has shown improvements in 3D reconstruction/registration/tracking. [11] proposed a more general solution using the Random Walks (RW) algorithm for US attenuation estimation and shadow detection. In their work, ultrasound confidence maps are obtained to classify the reliability of US intensity information, and thus, to detect regions of acoustic shadow. Their approach yields good results for 3D US compounding but is sensitive to US transducer settings. [12] further extended the RW method to generate distribution-based confidence maps for a specific Radio Frequency (RF) US data. Other applications, such as [4,6], use acoustic shadow detection as additional information in their pipeline. In both works, acoustic shadow detection functions as task-specific components, and is mainly based on image intensity features and the special anatomical constraints.

Advances in weakly supervised deep learning methods have drastically improved fully automatic semantic real-time image understanding [14,17,21]. However, most of these methods require pixel-wise labels for the training data, which is infeasible for acoustic shadows.

Unsupervised deep learning methods, showing visual attribution of different classes, have recently been developed in the context of Alzheimer's disease classification from MRI brain scans [3].

Inspired by these works, we develop a method to identify potential shadow areas based on supervised classification of weakly labelled, anatomically-focused US images, and further extend the detection of potential shadow areas using the visual attribution from an unsupervised model. We then combine intensity features, extracted by a graph-cut model, with potential shadow areas to provide a pixel-wise, shadow-focused confidence map. The overview of the proposed method is shown in Fig. 1.

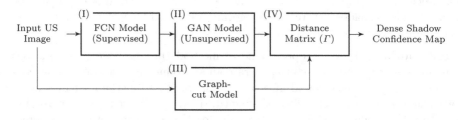

Fig. 1. Pipeline of the proposed method. (I) Identify potential shadow areas by a FCN model; (II) Extend obtained potential shadow areas using a GAN model; (III) Graph-cut is used to extract intensity features; (IV) The proposed distance matrix is designed to generate dense shadow confidence map from potential shadow areas and intensity features.

2   Method

Figure 2 shows an detailed inference flowchart over our method, which consists of four steps: (I) and (II) are used to highlight potential shadow areas, while step (III) selects coarse shadow areas based on intensity information. (IV) combines detection results from (II) and (III) to achieve the final shadow confidence map.

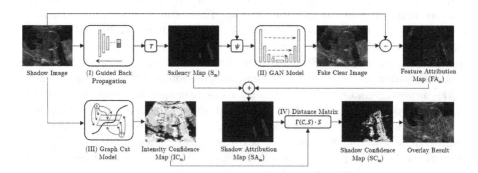

Fig. 2. Inference of our anatomy agnostic shadow detection approach.

(I) Saliency Map Generation: Saliency maps are generated by finding discriminative features from a trained classifier, using a gradient based back-propagation method, and thus, highlight distinct areas among different classes. Based on this property, it is a naïve approach to use saliency maps generated by shadow/shadow-free classifier for shadow detection.

We use a Fully Convolutional Neural-Network (FCN) to discern images containing shadows from shadow-free images. Here, we denote the has-shadow class with label $l = 1$ and the shadow-free class with label $l = 0$. Image set $X = \{x_1, x_2, ..., x_K\}$ and their corresponding labels $L = \{l_1, l_2, ..., l_K\}$ s.t. $l_i \in \{0, 1\}$ are used to train the FCN. The classifier provides predictions $p(x_i | l = 1)$ for image x_i during testing. We build the classifier model using SonoNet-32 [2], as it has shown promising results for 2D ultrasound fetal standard view classification. The training of the classifier is shown in Fig. 3.

Based on the trained shadow/shadow-free classifier, corresponding saliency maps $S_m = [s_{m1}, s_{m2}, ..., s_{mN}]$ are generated by guided back-propagation [19] for N testing samples. Shadows typically have features such as directional occlusion with relatively low intensity. These features, highlighted in S_m, are potential shadow candidates on a per-pixel basis.

However, by using gradient based back-propagation, saliency maps may ignore some areas which are evidence of a class but may have no ultimate effect on the classification result. In the shadow detection task, obtained saliency maps focus mainly on the edge of shadow areas but may ignore the homogeneous centre of shadow areas.

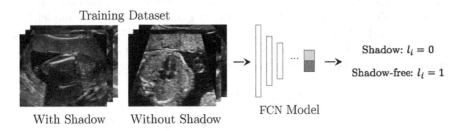

Fig. 3. Training FCN model for saliency map (S_m) generation

(II) Potential Shadow Areas Detection: Saliency maps heavily favour edges of the largest shadow region, especially when the image has multiple shadows, because these areas are the main difference between shadow and shadow-free images. In order to detect more shadows and inspired by VA-GAN [3], we develop a GAN model (shown in Fig. 4) that utilizes S_m to generate a Shadow Attribution Map (SA_m). S_m is used to inpaint the corresponding shadow image before passing the shadow image into the GAN model, so that the GAN model is forced to focus on other distinct areas between shadow and shadow-free images. Compared to S_m alone, this GAN model allows detection of more edges of relatively weak shadow areas as well as central areas of shadows.

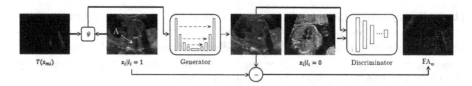

Fig. 4. Training GAN model for Feature Attribution map (FA_m) Generation.

The generator of the GAN model, G, produces a fake clear image from a shadow image x_i that has been inpainted with a binary mask of its corresponding saliency map. G has a U-Net structure with all its convolution layers being replaced by residual-units [9]. We optimize G by the Wasserstein distance [1], as it simplifies the optimization process and makes training more stable. The discriminator of the GAN model, D, is used to discern fake clear images from real clear images, and is trained with unpaired data. In the proposed method, the discriminator is a FCN without dense layers.

The inpainting function, used for the GAN input, is defined as $\psi := \psi(x_i|l_i = 1, T(s_{mi}))$. Here, $T_b^a(\cdot)$ produces a pixel-wise binary mask to identify pixels that lie in the top a and bottom b percentile of the input's intensity histogram distribution. In our experiments, we take the 2nd and 98th percentile respectively of the saliency map, s.t. $T_2^{98}(s_{mi}) = \{0 : P_2 \le s_{mi} \le P_{98}, 1 : \text{otherwise}\}$. ψ then replaces pixels in $x_i(T_2^{98}(s_{mi}) = 1)$ with the mean intensity value of $x_i(T_2^{98}(s_{mi}) = 0)$. The generator therefore focuses on more ambiguous shadow areas, as well as the central areas of shadows, to generate the fake clear image.

The overall cost function (shown in Eq. 1) consists of the GAN model loss $\mathcal{L}_{GAN}(G, D)$, a L1-loss $\mathcal{L}_1$ and a L2-loss $\mathcal{L}_2$. The $\mathcal{L}_{GAN}(G, D)$ is defined in Eq. 2. $\mathcal{L}_1$ is defined as in Eq. 3 to guarantee small changes in the output, while $\mathcal{L}_2$ is defined as Eq. 4 to encourage changes to happen only in potential shadow areas.

$$\mathcal{L} = \mathcal{L}_{GAN}(G, D) + \lambda_1 \mathcal{L}_1 + \lambda_2 \mathcal{L}_2 \tag{1}$$

$$\mathcal{L}_{GAN}(G, D) = \mathbf{E}_{\psi(\cdot) \sim p(\psi(\cdot)|l=0)}[D(x_i)] - \mathbf{E}_{\psi(\cdot) \sim p(\psi(\cdot)|l=1)}[D(G(\psi(\cdot)))] \tag{2}$$

$$\mathcal{L}_1 = ||G(\psi(\cdot)) - \psi(\cdot)||_1 \tag{3}$$

$$\mathcal{L}_2 = ||G(\psi(\cdot)_B - \psi(\cdot)_B||_2 \tag{4}$$

We train the networks using the optimisation method from [8] and set the gradient penalty as 10. The parameters for the optimiser are $\beta_1 = 0$, $\beta_2 = 0.9$, with the learning rate 10^{-3}. In the first 30 iterations and every hundredth iteration, the discriminator updates 100 times for every update of the generator. In other iterations, the discriminator updates five times for every single update of the generator. We set the weights of the combined loss function to $\lambda_1 = 0, \lambda_2 = 0.1$ for the first 20 epochs and $\lambda_1 = 10^4, \lambda_2 = 0$ for the remaining epochs.

The Feature Attribution map, FA_m, defined in Eq. 5, is obtained by subtracting the generated fake clear image from the original shadow image. The Shadow Attribution map is then $SA_m = FA_m + S_m$.

$$FA_m = |G(\psi(x_i|l_i = 1, T(s_{mi}))) - x_i| \tag{5}$$

(III) Graph Cut Model: Another feature of shadows is their relatively low intensity. To integrate this feature, we build a graph cut model using intensity information as weights to connect each pixel in the image to shadow class and background class. After using the Min-Cut/Max-Flow algorithm [20] to cut the graph, the model shows pixels belonging to the shadow class. The weights that connect pixels to the shadow class give an intensity saliency map IC_m.

Since shadow ground truth is not available for every image, we randomly select ten shadow images from training data for manual segmentation to compute the shadow mean intensity I_S. Background mean intensity I_B is computed by thresholding these ten images using the top 80th percentile.

For a pixel x_{ij} with intensity I_{ij}, the score of being a shadow pixel F_{ij} is given by Eq. 6 while the score of being a background pixel B_{ij} is given by Eq. 7. The weight from x_{ij} to source (shadow class) is set as $W_{F_{ij}} = \frac{F_{ij}}{F_{ij}+B_{ij}}$ and the weight from x_{ij} to sink (background) is $W_{B_{ij}} = \frac{B_{ij}}{F_{ij}+B_{ij}}$. We use a 4-connected neighbourhood to set weights between pixels and all the weights between neighbourhood pixels are set to 0.5.

$$F_{ij} = -\frac{|I_{ij} - I_S|}{|I_{ij} - I_S| + |I_{ij} - I_B|} \tag{6}$$

$$B_{ij} = -\frac{|I_{ij} - I_B|}{|I_{ij} - I_S| + |I_{ij} - I_B|} \tag{7}$$

(IV) Distance Matrix: Since the intensity distribution of shadow areas are homogeneous, potential shadow areas detected in SA_m from (II) are mainly edges of shadows. Meanwhile, IC_m from (III) shows all pixels with a similar intensity to shadow areas. In this step, we propose a distance matrix $\mathbf{D}$ combining IC_m with SA_m to produce a Shadow Confidence Map (SC_m). In SC_m, pixels with a similar intensity to shadow areas and spatially closer to potential shadow areas achieves higher confidence of being part of shadow areas.

$$\Gamma(IC_m, SA_m) = 1 - \frac{Dis}{\max(Dis)} \tag{8}$$

$$SC_m = \Gamma(IC_m, SA_m) \cdot IC_m \tag{9}$$

The distance matrix is defined in Eq. 8. Dis is the set of the spatial distances that each pixel IC_{mij} to potential shadow areas in SA_m. Each element Dis_{ij} in Dis refers to the smallest distance of IC_{mij} to all connected components in SA_m. SC_m is obtained by multiplying the distance matrix Γ to IC_m (shown in Eq. 9) which leads to pixels with similar shadow area intensity and closer to the potential shadow areas achieve a higher score in SC_m.

3   Evaluation and Results

US Image Data: The data set used in our experiments consists of ~8.5k 2D fetal ultrasound images sampled from 14 different anatomical standard plane locations as they are defined in the UK FASP handbook [16]. These images have been sampled from 2694 2D ultrasound examinations from volunteers with gestational ages between 18–22 weeks. Eight different ultrasound systems of identical make and model (GE Voluson E8) were used for the acquisitions. The images have been classified by expert observers as containing strong shadow, being clear, or being corrupted, e.g. lacking acoustic impedance gel. Corrupted images (<3%) have been excluded.

3448 shadow images and 3842 clear images have been randomly selected for data set **A**, which is used for training. The remaining 491 shadow images and 502 clear images are used for validation. Data set **B**, a subset from the 491 shadow validation images, comprises of 48 randomly selected non-brain images, where shadows have been manually segmented to provide ground truth.

An additional data set **C**, which has no overlap with the ~8.5k fetal images, comprises of 643 fetal brain images. The entire data set C has been used for validation and shadows in this data set been coarsely segmented by bioengineering students.

We apply image flipping as data augmentation. Our models are trained on a Nvidia Titan X GPU with 12 GB of memory.

Table 1. Threshold ranges and DICE scores of different shadow detection methods: RW [11] vs. intermediate results from our approach and the final shadow confidence map.

	RW	S_m	FA_m	SA_m	**SC_m**
Dataset B	$T_3^{100}(S_m)$	$T_1^{99}(S_m)$	$T_1^{85}(FA_m)$	$T_1^{96}(SA_m)$	$T_0^{80}(SC_m)$
	0.06	0.25	0.06	0.27	**0.55**
Dataset C	$T_3^{100}(S_m)$	$T_1^{99}(S_m)$	$T_1^{80}(FA_m)$	$T_0^{90}(SA_m)$	$T_0^{70}(SC_m)$
	0.11	0.28	0.08	0.31	**0.36**

Experiment Results: The classification accuracy of the FCN classifier on the validation data set C is 94%. The FCN classifier's saliency maps are shown in Fig. 5 column (b) for three examples from data set B and C.

To provide quantitative evaluation (Table 1), we chose the percentile range used by T for SC_m as well as other intermediate maps (S_m, FA_m, SA_m). These percentile ranges for different maps are chosen heuristically through experimentations on validation data set B and C, so that these thresholded segmentation of data set B and C contains the most shadow areas and the least noise. We compare these thresholded segmentation with manual segmentation in data set B and C using the DICE score. Additionally, we compare the thresholded versions of the confidence map derived from the RW method [11]. The parameters for RW

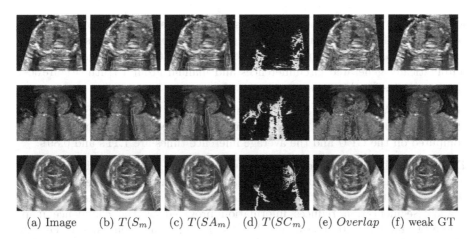

(a) Image   (b) $T(S_m)$ (c) $T(SA_m)$ (d) $T(SC_m)$ (e) *Overlap*   (f) weak GT

Fig. 5. Rows 1–3 show examples for shadow detection; Right Ventricular Outflow Tract (top), Kidney (middle), and an axial view through the brain (bottom). The key steps from Fig. 2 are illustrated from (a) the input image to (f) the coarse ground truth (GT) from manual segmentation.

in our experiments are: $\alpha = 1$; $\beta = 90$; $\gamma = 0.3$, which reach the highest DICE score on our validation data sets. Qualitative results are shown in Fig. 5. The GAN model in our approach is essential as it picks up less prominent shadows as shown in Fig. 6.

Application: We integrate SC_m as an additional channel in a clinical system that automatically measures cranial and abdominal circumferences [18]. This system is based on FCNs and works well for images without shadows but fails

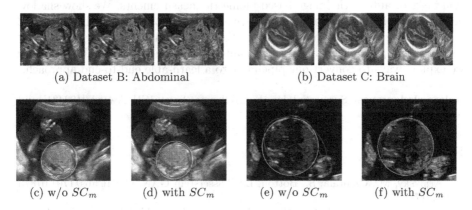

(a) Dataset B: Abdominal   (b) Dataset C: Brain

(c) w/o SC_m (d) with SC_m (e) w/o SC_m (f) with SC_m

Fig. 6. (a–b) Two examples for the importance of the GAN model (input image – w/o GAN – with GAN). (c–f) Improving automatic biometric measurements through applying SC_m as additional channel to a FCN [18] (yellow = GT, red = prediction, green = segmentation boundary). (Color figure online)

for about 5–10% of abdominal test images which show strong shadows. By adding SC_m as an additional input channel, segmentation performance is boosted by up to 10% for individual failure cases, when measuring the DICE overlap between automatically generated circumferences and manual ground truth. Figure 5c–f show examples for these cases.

Runtime: IC_m, SA_m and SC_m are computed on the CPU (Xeon E5-2643) and the average runtimes are 1.86 s, 0.09 s and 7.4 s respectively. S_m and FA_m are computed on the GPU and the average inference times are 1.11 s and 0.89 s.

Discussion: Because shadow areas have no solid edges and can be harder to annotated consistently than anatomy, manual segmentation can be ambiguous. Additionally, thresholding the shadow confidence map to generate a binary shadow segmentation reduces information provided by the confidence map. These two facts lead to a seemingly low DICE score when compared to current object segmentation frameworks. However, shadows are image properties rather than objects, and our final aim is to provide a confidence map, which cannot be compared quantitatively to a ground truth. The quantitative measurement in Table 1 indicates the effectiveness of the proposed method compared with the state-of-the-art method when handling complex shadow images. The qualitative results in Fig. 5 show accurate shadow detection of the proposed method and Fig. 6 demonstrate the importance of shadow detection in automatic medical image analysis.

4   Conclusion

We have presented a novel method to generate pixel-wise, shadow-focused confidence maps for 2D ultrasound. Such confidence maps can be used to identify less certain regions in images, which is important for fully automatic segmentation tasks or automatic image-based biometric measurements. We show shadow detection results of our method qualitatively and compare our method with the state-of-the-art method quantitatively. We also show the advantage of shadow confidence maps via integration into an automatic biometrics FCN. In the future we explore ways to convert our pipeline into a learn-able end-to-end approach.

Acknowledgments. Supported by the Wellcome Trust IEH Award [102431] and Nvidia Corporation.

References

1. Arjovsky, M., Chintala, S., Bottou, L.: Wasserstein GAN. CoRR abs/1701.07875 (2017)
2. Baumgartner, C., et al.: SonoNet: real-time detection and localisation of fetal standard scan planes in freehand ultrasound. IEEE Trans. Med. Imaging **36**(11), 2204–2215 (2017)
3. Baumgartner, C., Koch, L., Tezcan, K., Ang, J., Konukoglu, E.: Visual feature attribution using Wasserstein GANs. CoRR abs/1711.08998 (2017)

4. Berton, F., Cheriet, F., Miron, M.-C., Laporte, C.: Segmentation of the spinous process and its acoustic shadow in vertebral ultrasound images. Comput. Biol. Med. **72**, 201–211 (2016)
5. Bouhemad, B., Zhang, M., Lu, Q., Rouby, J.: Clinical review: bedside lung ultrasound in critical care practice. Crit. Care **11**(1), 205 (2007)
6. Broersen, A., et al.: Enhanced characterization of calcified areas in intravascular ultrasound virtual histology images by quantification of the acoustic shadow: validation against computed tomography coronary angiography. Int. J. Cardiovasc. Imaging **32**, 543–552 (2015)
7. Coupé, P., Hellier, P., Kervrann, C., Barillot, C.: Nonlocal means-based speckle filtering for ultrasound images. IEEE Trans. Image Process. **18**(10), 2221–2229 (2009)
8. Gulrajani, I., Ahmed, F., Arjovsky, M., Dumoulin, V., Courville, A.: Improved training of Wasserstein GANs. CoRR abs/1704.00028 (2017)
9. He, K., Zhang, X., Ren, S., Sun, J.: Identity mappings in deep residual networks. In: Leibe, B., Matas, J., Sebe, N., Welling, M. (eds.) ECCV 2016. LNCS, vol. 9908, pp. 630–645. Springer, Cham (2016). https://doi.org/10.1007/978-3-319-46493-0_38
10. Hellier, P., Coupé, P., Morandi, X., Collins, D.: An automatic geometrical and statistical method to detect acoustic shadows in intraoperative ultrasound brain images. Med. Image Anal. **14**(2), 195–204 (2010)
11. Karamalis, A., Wein, W., Klein, T., Navab, N.: Ultrasound confidence maps using random walks. Med. Image Anal. **16**(6), 1101–1112 (2012)
12. Klein, T., Wells, W.M.: RF ultrasound distribution-based confidence maps. In: Navab, N., Hornegger, J., Wells, W.M., Frangi, A.F. (eds.) MICCAI 2015. LNCS, vol. 9350, pp. 595–602. Springer, Cham (2015). https://doi.org/10.1007/978-3-319-24571-3_71
13. Kremkau, F.W., Taylor, K.: Artifacts in ultrasound imaging. J. Ultrasound Med. **5**(4), 227–237 (1986)
14. Krizhevsky, A., Sutskever, I., Hinton, G.: ImageNet classification with deep convolutional neural networks. In: NIPS 2012, pp. 1097–1105 (2012)
15. Lange, T., et al.: 3D ultrasound-CT registration of the liver using combined landmark-intensity information. Int. J. Comput. Assist. Radiol. Surg. **4**(1), 79–88 (2009)
16. NHS: Fetal anomaly screening programme: programme handbook June 2015. Public Health England (2015)
17. Rajchl, M., et al.: DeepCut: object segmentation from bounding box annotations using convolutional neural networks. IEEE Trans. Med. Imaging **36**(2), 674–683 (2017)
18. Sinclair, M., et al.: Human-level performance on automatic head biometrics in fetal ultrasound using fully convolutional neural networks. In: EMBC 2018 (2018)
19. Springenberg, J., Dosovitskiy, A., Brox, T., Riedmiller, M.: Striving for simplicity: the all convolutional net. CoRR abs/1412.6806 (2014)
20. Yuri, B., Vladimir, K.: An experimental comparison of min-cut/max-flow algorithms for energy minimization in vision. IEEE Trans. Pattern Anal. Mach. Intell. **26**(9), 1124–1137 (2004)
21. Zhou, B., Khosla, A., Lapedriza, A., Oliva, A., Torralba, A.: Learning deep features for discriminative localization. In: CVPR 2016, pp. 2921–2929. IEEE (2016)

Multi-channel Groupwise Registration to Construct an Ultrasound-Specific Fetal Brain Atlas

Ana I. L. Namburete[1(✉)], Raquel van Kampen[1], Aris T. Papageorghiou[2], and Bartłomiej W. Papież[1,3]

[1] Institute of Biomedical Engineering, Department of Engineering Science,
University of Oxford, Oxford, UK
ana.namburete@eng.ox.ac.uk
[2] Nuffield Department of Obstetrics and Gynaecology, John Radcliffe Hospital,
University of Oxford, Oxford, UK
[3] Big Data Institute, Li Ka Shing Centre for Health Information and Discovery,
University of Oxford, Oxford, UK

Abstract. In this paper, we describe a method to construct a 3D atlas from fetal brain ultrasound (US) volumes. A multi-channel groupwise Demons registration is proposed to simultaneously register a set of images from a population to a common reference space, thereby representing the population average. Similar to the standard Demons formulation, our approach takes as input an intensity image, but with an additional channel which contains phase-based features extracted from the intensity channel. The proposed multi-channel atlas construction method is evaluated using a groupwise Dice overlap, and is shown to outperform standard (single-channel) groupwise diffeomorphic Demons registration. This method is then used to construct an atlas from US brain volumes collected from a population of 39 healthy fetal subjects at 23 gestational weeks. The resulting atlas manifests high structural overlap, and correspondence between the US-based and an age-matched fetal MRI-based atlas is observed.

1 Introduction

Tracking fetal growth and developmental progression is paramount in obstetric care. The fetal brain undergoes a predictable sequence of structural changes across gestation: from a smooth surface, to progressively bearing more folds [1]. This process follows a precise schedule, and delays are indicative of impaired brain maturation. Thus, the presence of a cerebral abnormality may be manifested by structural deviations from the norm. In order to detect such developmental deviations, an individual's image can be compared against an atlas that is representative of the healthy population. Atlases of the developing brain have been developed from magnetic resonance (MR) image data collected from infant and fetal subjects (reviewed in [2]). These atlases have provided a representation of brain anatomy in the womb, and have facilitated tissue segmentation, thereby

© Springer Nature Switzerland AG 2018
A. Melbourne and R. Licandro et al. (Eds.): DATRA/PIPPI 2018, LNCS 11076, pp. 76–86, 2018.
https://doi.org/10.1007/978-3-030-00807-9_8

enabling studies of structural growth and aiding the detection (or characteri-zation) of fetal pathologies [2]. However, given that ultrasound (US) imaging forms one of the first steps in perinatal monitoring, there is still a need to create an *ultrasound-specific* atlas for use in routine care. This work presents a tool to automatically generate an atlas from 3D US images of the fetal brain.

The standard approach to construct an anatomical atlas is to perform one of state-of-the-art pairwise deformable registration algorithms [3] between the chosen (reference) volume and the remaining volumes from a data set. Such an approach is simple and easily scalable to large data sets, however it introduces a bias to registration results due to the selection of reference volume. That is, if the selected reference volume is an outlier then all registrations will estimate implausible transformations. Additionally, the transformation estimated using a pairwise approach accumulates inverse consistency and transitivity errors [4], which could be propagated to any subsequent analysis. Different approaches have been proposed to reduce transformation errors when building atlases, including statistical deformation models [5], linear [6] or geodesic [7,8] averaging of the transformations and intensity to produce the atlases. Approaches with simulta-neous registration (i.e. *groupwise registration*) of all volumes in a dataset have been shown to reduce the bias introduced by selection of a fixed reference volume, and errors in the estimated displacement fields.

Developing intensity-based methods for registration of ultrasound images is challenging due to strong intensity inhomogeneities within tissues, and the pres-ence of shadows, which cause partial, low-contrast boundaries. Local phase [9] and feature asymmetry (derived from the monogenic signal [10]) extract contrast-invariant structural information, and have been shown to improve analysis of US images in several tasks. Specifically, feature asymmetry (FA) has the potential to enhance tissue boundaries, and as such, has been extensively used to process fetal ultrasound data, where there are large structural changes (e.g. [11,12]). A hybrid intensity and local phase representation of US images has been applied to tumour tracking in 2D liver US [13], showing overall improved registration accuracy. Realizing the potential of FA to enhance and sharpen the sonographic landmarks necessary for accurate registration, this work explores its inclusion as additional image channels for US atlas construction.

In this paper, we present a framework to construct the first 3D atlas of the fetal brain using non-rigid groupwise registration of US images. Our framework extends a standard groupwise registration [4] to its multi-channel counterpart using a composite image representation to improve the registration of tissue interfaces in US data. The proposed multi-channel image representation com-prises of ultrasound intensities and features extracted using different FA scales, thereby representing boundaries of different sizes in a multiscale manner. The presented evaluation shows that the presented method is capable of constructing an atlas from fetal brain US data, and at the same time, the performed quan-titative analysis shows that our method outperforms standard intensity-based, and single channel image registration methods.

2   Materials and Methods

2.1   Fetal Dataset and Preprocessing

The fetal US images used in this work comprised of 39 volumes ($247 \times 190 \times 179$ voxels) with known age of 23 gestational weeks (GW). The sonographic volumes of the fetal head were obtained from the INTERGROWTH-21st study database [14], which were collected using a Philips HD9 curvilinear probe at a 2–5 MHz wave frequency. After alignment [15], all volumes were resampled to an isotropic voxel size ($0.6 \times 0.6 \times 0.6$ mm) and resized to $160 \times 160 \times 160$ voxels.

2.2   Atlas Construction

Given a set of M images, the goal of atlas construction is to find a set of transformations $\mathcal{T}$, each of which maps its corresponding image $\mathbf{I}_m$ to a common reference space: $\mathcal{T} : \{\boldsymbol{T}_{mR} : \mathbf{I}_m \mapsto \mathbf{I}_R, m = 1, \ldots, M\}$. This typically comprises of two steps: a global transformation to correct for size and growth differences, followed by a non-rigid registration to account for local morphological differences.

Sonographic scans of the fetal head were first rigidly aligned using the method proposed in [15]. Briefly, a slice-wise classifier segmented the skull boundaries and predicted the relative position of the slice in the brain volume. This information was then combined to estimate a similarity transformation modelling 9 degrees of freedom (namely, rotation, translation, and isotropic scaling) to linearly register all volumes to a standard (atlas) space. One of the challenges of processing fetal brain US is that the ultrasound signal is attenuated by the cranial bones in its path, and the concave shape also refracts it and creates reverberation artifacts. This affects the visibility of anatomical boundaries, particularly in the cerebral hemisphere proximal to the US probe. Since only one of the hemispheres has clearly visible structures, this hemisphere is mirrored across the midsagittal plane. This generates a *complete* representation of the brain, thereby making an assumption of brain symmetry, for simplicity [16].

The non-rigid image registration used in this work, is built on the groupwise deformable registration proposed in [4,17]. The implicit reference groupwise registration reduces bias introduced by selection of a reference volume by jointly estimating the transformation between all volumes in the dataset to an *unknown* reference volume. This process is defined as the following optimization problem:

$$\arg\min_{\boldsymbol{u}} \left(\sum_m^M \sum_{n,n\neq m}^M \int_\Omega Sim\left(\mathbf{I}_m(\boldsymbol{T}_{mR}(\boldsymbol{x})), \mathbf{I}_n(\boldsymbol{T}_{nR}(\boldsymbol{x}))\right) d\boldsymbol{x} + \tag{1}$$

$$\alpha \sum_m^M \int_\Omega Reg(\boldsymbol{u}_{mR}(\boldsymbol{x})) d\boldsymbol{x} \right) \tag{2}$$

where Sim and Reg denote the similarity measure and regularisation term, respectively, α is the weighting parameter, $\boldsymbol{T}_{mR} = \boldsymbol{x} + \boldsymbol{u}_{mR}(\boldsymbol{x})$ (or $\boldsymbol{T}_{nR} =$

$x + u_{nR}(x))$ is the transformation from volume $\mathbf{I}_m$ (or $\mathbf{I}_n$) to the implicit reference volume $\mathbf{I}_R$ at spatial position x. The u_{mR} (or u_{nR}) represents a subsequent displacement field, Ω is the volume domain, and M is the number of volumes to be registered. The *implicit* reference volume is iteratively updated based on all the volumes deformed during the displacement field estimation process. In this work, we choose the diffeomorphic Demons framework [18], where optimisation iteratively alternates between minimising the energy related to the similarity measure *Sim* and the regularization term *Reg* performed via Gaussian smoothing of the estimated displacement fields. In order to establish anatomically meaningful correspondences between brain US volumes, we replace state-of-the-art intensity differences used in the classic Demons by a multi-channel feature-based representation of the US volumes. The implementation details for efficient Demons-like implicit reference groupwise registration can be found in [19].

2.3   Feature Extraction

The monogenic signal uses the Riesz transform to generate a representation of an image in the frequency domain [20]. By applying an appropriately selected bandpass filter ($f_{\{o,e\}}$), the signal can be decomposed into local structural (phase and orientation) and energetic (amplitude) information. The phase component extracts contrast-invariant, structural information, which is particularly useful in recovering feature asymmetry (FA) [21]. FA is a measure of the extent to which a structure around an image voxel is locally *asymmetric*, thus representing a step-edge [10,21]. The FA edge image $\hat{\mathbf{I}}$ of an input image $\mathbf{I}$ is recovered as:

$$\hat{\mathbf{I}} = \frac{\lfloor |f_{o,\lambda}(\mathbf{I})| - |f_{e,\lambda}(\mathbf{I})| - t \rfloor}{\sqrt{f_{o,\lambda}(\mathbf{I})^2 + f_{e,\lambda}(\mathbf{I})^2} + \varepsilon} \tag{3}$$

where λ represents the filter scale, f_o and f_e represent the odd and even parts of the signal, t is a threshold that controls the sensitivity of the response, $\lfloor \cdot \rfloor$ sets negative values to zero, and ε is a filter regularization parameter which prevents division by zero.

FA allows edge features to be obtained at different centre-wavelengths, λ. The centre frequency is equivalent to the scale of the bandpass filter $f_{\{o,e\},\lambda}$ (i.e. size of structures of interest) used to the calculate the monogenic signal. In fetal brain US images, the anatomical boundaries appear as step-edges and ridge-like structures, which are best extracted with a log-Gabor filter [11]. Given an US image, $\mathbf{I}$, a corresponding FA edge image $\hat{\mathbf{I}}$ is defined to highlight structural boundaries [10,21]. An FA image typically detects thick edges which are thinned by applying non-maximum suppression for improved boundary localization. Here, we explore the effect of supplementary structural information for atlas construction by varying the centre frequency at which the monogenic signal was recovered from the images, $\lambda = [0.025, 0.425]$ (Fig. 1). The other parameters were empirically set to $t = 0.5$ and $\varepsilon = 10^{-6}$.

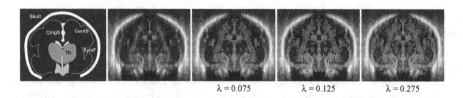

Fig. 1. Schematic of a coronal view of the fetal brain at 23 GW, and a typical US scan. Feature asymmetry edge images are shown at varying centre-frequency wavelengths, $\lambda = \{0.075, 0.125, 0.275\}$, overlaid in yellow. (Color figure online)

2.4   Evaluation Metrics

Ten brain volumes were linearly registered using [15] and anatomical regions were manually segmented and verified by an expert with 10 years' experience and a senior sonographer. The segmented regions of interest ($\mathbf{V}^k$) included the brain stem (BS), cavum septum pellucidum (CSP), thalamus (TH), and white matter (WM) (Fig. 2c). In order to evaluate registration performance, we compute the average relative overlap (ARO) for each of the $K = 4$ regions as follows [4]:

$$ARO = \frac{1}{N(N-1)} \sum_{\substack{j=1,\\ j \neq i}}^{N} \sum_{i=1}^{N} \frac{\sum_K \mathbf{V}_i^k \cap \mathbf{V}_j^k}{\sum_K \mathbf{V}_i^k \cup \mathbf{V}_j^k} \tag{4}$$

where $\mathbf{V}_i^k = \mathbf{V}_i^k \left(\mathcal{T}_{iR}(\mathbf{I}) \right)$, K is the number structures, and N is the number of annotated volumes.

All experiments were performed on an Intel i7 2.80 GHz quad-core machine (32 GB RAM) with a C++ implementation of the diffeomorphic Demons algorithm.

3   Results and Discussion

3.1   Registration of Anatomical Structures

In the first experiment, we explored different formulations of the groupwise registration algorithm to construct an atlas that maximizes anatomical correspondence between the neurosonographic images. By varying the diffusion parameter of the Demons-like forces ($\sigma_d = [0.25, 5.0]$), we find that the best performance is achieved with $\sigma_d = 1.0$ (ARO > 0.868 for WM, Fig. 2a), and gradually decreases as σ_d increases. This behaviour was observed regardless of input: single- or multi-channel.

Furthermore, we explored the effect of FA wavelength (scale) selection by varying λ from 0.025 to 0.425. Figure 2b shows the ARO averaged across all four structures. The groupwise approach outperformed the linearly aligned data, regardless of input. However, the multi-channel Demons (intensity + sFA) outperformed single-channel Demons (intensity) only for scales $\lambda = \{0.075, 0.125, 0.175\}$.

For further comparison, we explored the performance of a multi-channel Demons with multi-scale feature extraction by combining the features from the best FA scales ($\lambda = 0.075, 0.125, 0.175$) into the second input channel. This yielded the highest structural overlap (ARO = 0.8029 ± 0.049) and was selected as the best method for atlas construction.

Figure 2c shows the result of applying the groupwise registration to the set of ten volumes for which corresponding segmentations were available. The atlases were constructed by averaging the images after affine registration, and then further transformed by the groupwise registration. There is high consensus between the structures, as observed in the probability maps, which is corroborated by the groupwise ARO of the resulting atlas (Table 1).

To further examine the anatomical agreement recovered by the groupwise registration algorithm, we compared the average segmentation maps obtained by transforming the annotated images, with a segmentation of the resulting groupwise atlas. High volumetric overlap was also observed for all four structures (mean ARO = 0.8580 ± 0.036).

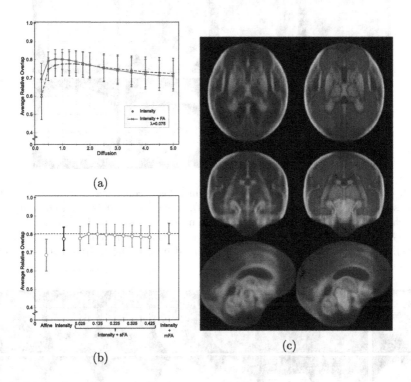

Fig. 2. (a) Registration regularization parameter (σ_d) versus average relative overlap (ARO). (b) Different atlas construction methods plotted against ARO. (c) Resulting US atlas constructed using intensity and multi-scale FA from $n = 10$ volumes for which segmentations were available. Denser colour signifies higher overlap.

3.2   Construction of Population Brain Atlas

In the second experiment, we applied the proposed multi-channel groupwise registration algorithm to 39 brain volumes to construct an atlas. Figure 3 shows atlases constructed by averaging the images after the affine registration [15], and after non-rigid registration with either a single (intensity) channel, or multiple channels (i.e. intensity and feature asymmetry). It is evident that the atlases constructed with groupwise registration had higher anatomical definition, and more distinct boundaries. Structural clarity was even higher in the atlas constructed with multi-channel inputs.

In order to visualize the structural variation within the healthy fetal cohort at 23 GW, we performed principal component analysis (PCA) of the deformation fields estimated from the 39 volumes. Figure 5 demonstrates the first four

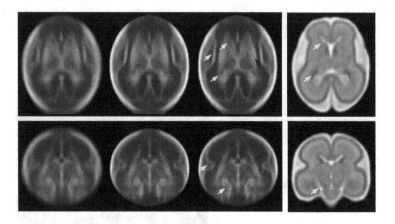

Fig. 3. Visual comparison between fetal brain atlases constructed from $n = 39$ US volumes at 23 GW using affine (first column), intensity-based (second column), and multi-channel groupwise methods (third column). Comparison to MRI-based fetal atlas at 23 GW shows the presence of similar structures in both modalities [22] (yellow arrows), but some structures are better observed in US images (red arrows). (Color figure online)

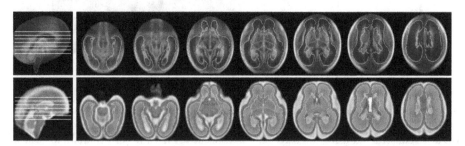

Fig. 4. Volumetric US atlas with superimposed segmentation of four structures from a fetal MR atlas at 23 GW (obtained from Gholipour et al. [22]).

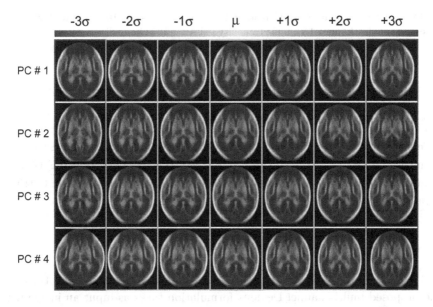

Fig. 5. Principal component analysis (PCA) result display the mean brain ±3 standard deviations (i.e. $\mu \pm 3\sigma$) for the first four components. All modes show realistic representations of the brain.

components, altogether explaining 65.6% of the variation at this gestational age. PC1, PC2, and PC4 display variations in anatomical shape and global eccentricity of the brain. Small changes in ventricular shape are particularly observed around the posterior lateral ventricles and the cortical plate in PC1. Nonetheless, all modes of variation demonstrate realistic representations of the brain at 23 GW.

3.3   Comparison to Existing Fetal Atlas

In order to assess the quality of the resulting atlas, Fig. 4 compares our US-specific atlas with a MRI-based fetal template at 23 GW generated by Gholipour et al. [22]. The contours of the latter are superimposed on the US-based atlas constructed from $n = 39$ volumes. Here, we can visually determine that despite there not being a direct intensity mapping between the two, there is a good match between the shape and location of the structures in both modalities at this gestational week. This illustrates the complementarity between the modalities, and presents opportunities to transfer anatomical insights from one to the other, and the possibility to facilitate analysis of fetal brain US with information contained within MRI models of development (e.g. [22]). The fact that structures such as the basal ganglia are better visible in the US-based atlas (Fig. 3) also presents new opportunities for use of neurosonographic data to study structural development.

Table 1. Average relative overlap for all four structures on 10 annotated volumes. Intensity: single-channel Demons. Intensity+sFA: multi-channel, single-scale demons ($\lambda = 0.075$). Intensity+mFA: multi-channel, multi-scale Demons with FA scales $\lambda = \{0.075, 0.125, 0.175\}$.

Method	Structural ARO ($\bar{D}^k$)				Mean ARO
	WM	TH	CSP	BS	
Linear only [15]	0.8174	0.6467	0.6379	0.6412	0.6858 ± 0.076
Intensity	0.8680	0.7383	0.7289	0.7652	0.7751 ± 0.055
Intensity + sFA	0.8829	0.7672	0.7806	**0.7771**	0.8019 ± 0.047
Intensity + mFA	**0.8873**	**0.7680**	**0.7824**	0.7738	$\mathbf{0.8029 \pm 0.049}$
Structural volume (cm^3)	37.64	1.954	0.449	1.233	–

4   Conclusion

In this paper, we present the first fetal brain atlas constructed from US data. The proposed multi-channel Demons formulation takes as input an image with intensity and feature-enhanced channels. It was shown to outperform a single-channel Demons registration approach, generating high structural overlap in the resulting atlas. Comparison with an age-matched MR atlas demonstrated similarities in the shape and presence of key anatomies in both imaging modalities, but also revealed new structures that are better observed in the US atlas. Given the formulation of the proposed method, it is expected that it should extend to a broader gestational age range.

Acknowledgements. A. Namburete is grateful for support from the Royal Academy of Engineering under the Engineering for Development Research Fellowship scheme. B. Papiez acknowledges Oxford NIHR Biomedical Research Centre (Rutherford Fund Fellowship at HDR UK). We thank the INTERGROWTH-21st and INTERBIO-21st Consortia for provision of 3D fetal US image data.

References

1. Toi, A., Lister, W.S., Fong, K.W.: How early are fetal cerebral sulci visible at prenatal ultrasound and what is the normal pattern of early fetal sulcal development? Ultrasound Obstet. Gynecol. **24**(7), 706–715 (2004)
2. Makropoulos, A., Counsell, S.J., Rueckert, D.: A review on automatic fetal and neonatal brain MRI segmentation. NeuroImage **170**, 231–248 (2018)
3. Sotiras, A., Davatzikos, C., Paragios, N.: Deformable medical image registration: a survey. IEEE Trans. Med. Imaging **32**(7), 1153–1190 (2013)
4. Geng, X., Christensen, G.E., Gu, H., Ross, T.J., Yang, Y.: Implicit reference-based group-wise image registration and its application to structural and functional MRI. NeuroImage **47**(4), 1341–1351 (2009)
5. Rueckert, D., Frangi, A.F., Schnabel, J.A.: Automatic construction of 3-D statistical deformation models of the brain using nonrigid registration. IEEE Trans. Med. Imaging **22**(8), 1014–1025 (2003)

6. Guimond, A., Meunier, J., Thirion, J.: Average brain models: a convergence study. Comput. Vis. Image Underst. **77**(2), 192–210 (2000)
7. Avants, B., Gee, J.C.: Geodesic estimation for large deformation anatomical shape averaging and interpolation. Neuroimage **23**, S139–S150 (2004)
8. Joshi, S., Davis, B., Jomier, M., Gerig, G.: Unbiased diffeomorphic atlas construction for computational anatomy. NeuroImage **23**, S151–S160 (2004)
9. Mellor, M., Brady, M.: Non-rigid multimodal image registration using local phase. In: Barillot, C., Haynor, D.R., Hellier, P. (eds.) MICCAI 2004. LNCS, vol. 3216, pp. 789–796. Springer, Heidelberg (2004). https://doi.org/10.1007/978-3-540-30135-6_96
10. Bridge, C.P.: Introduction to the monogenic signal. CoRR abs/1703.09199 (2017)
11. Namburete, A.I.L., Stebbing, R.V., Kemp, B., Yaqub, M., Papageorghiou, A.T., Alison Noble, J.: Learning-based prediction of gestational age from ultrasound images of the fetal brain. Med. Image Anal. **21**(1), 72–86 (2015)
12. Rueda, S., Knight, C.L., Papageorghiou, A.T., Noble, J.A.: Feature-based fuzzy connectedness segmentation of ultrasound images with an object completion step. Med. Image Anal. **26**(1), 30–46 (2015)
13. Cifor, A., Risser, L., Chung, D., Anderson, E.M., Schnabel, J.A.: Hybrid feature-based diffeomorphic registration for tumor tracking in 2-D liver ultrasound images. IEEE Trans. Med. Imaging **32**(9), 1647–1656 (2013)
14. Papageorghiou, A.T., et al.: International Fetal and Newborn Growth Consortium for the 21st Century (INTERGROWTH-21st): International standards for fetal growth based on serial ultrasound measurements: the Fetal Growth Longitudinal Study of the INTERGROWTH-21st Project. Lancet **384**(9946), 869–79 (2014)
15. Namburete, A.I., Xie, W., Yaqub, M., Zisserman, A., Noble, J.A.: Fully-automated alignment of 3D fetal brain ultrasound to a canonical reference space using multi-task learning. Med. Image Anal. **46**, 1–14 (2018)
16. Namburete, A.I.L., Xie, W., Noble, J.A.: Robust regression of brain maturation from 3D fetal neurosonography using CRNs. In: Cardoso, M.J., et al. (eds.) FIFI/OMIA -2017. LNCS, vol. 10554, pp. 73–80. Springer, Cham (2017). https://doi.org/10.1007/978-3-319-67561-9_8
17. Papiez, B.W., Matuszewski, B.J., Shark, L.K., Quan, W.: Facial expression recognition using diffeomorphic image registration framework. In: Latorre Carmona P., Sánchez J., Fred A. (eds.) Mathematical Methodologies in Pattern Recognition and Machine Learning. Springer Proceedings in Mathematics & Statistics, vol. 30. Springer, New York (2013). https://doi.org/10.1007/978-1-4614-5076-4_12
18. Vercauteren, T., Pennec, X., Perchant, A., Ayache, N.: Symmetric log-domain diffeomorphic registration: a demons-based approach. In: Metaxas, D., Axel, L., Fichtinger, G., Székely, G. (eds.) MICCAI 2008. LNCS, vol. 5241, pp. 754–761. Springer, Heidelberg (2008). https://doi.org/10.1007/978-3-540-85988-8_90
19. Papież, B.W., McGowan, D.R., Skwarski, M., Higgins, G.S., Schnabel, J.A., Brady, M.: Fast groupwise 4D deformable image registration for irregular breathing motion estimation. In: Klein, S., Staring, M., Durrleman, S., Sommer, S. (eds.) WBIR 2018. LNCS, vol. 10883, pp. 37–46. Springer, Cham (2018). https://doi.org/10.1007/978-3-319-92258-4_4
20. Felsberg, M., Sommer, G.: The monogenic signal. IEEE Trans. Sig. Process. **49**(12), 3136–3144 (2001)

21. Kovesi, P.: Invariant Measures of Image Features from Phase Information. Ph.D thesis, The University of Western Australia (1996)
22. Gholipour, A., et al.: A normative spatiotemporal MRI atlas of the fetal brain for automatic segmentation and analysis of early brain growth. Sci. Rep. **7**(1), 1 (2017)

Investigating Brain Age Deviation in Preterm Infants: A Deep Learning Approach

Susmita Saha[1]([⊠])🆔, Alex Pagnozzi[1]🆔, Joanne George[3]🆔,
Paul B. Colditz[2]🆔, Roslyn Boyd[3]🆔, Stephen Rose[1],
Jurgen Fripp[1]🆔, and Kerstin Pannek[1]🆔

[1] Australian E-Health Research Centre, CSIRO, Brisbane, Australia
susmita.saha@csiro.au
[2] Centre for Clinical Research, Faculty of Medicine,
The University of Queensland, Brisbane, Australia
[3] Queensland Cerebral Palsy and Rehabilitation Research Centre,
Centre for Children's Health Research, Faculty of Medicine,
The University of Queensland, Brisbane, Australia

Abstract. This study examined postmenstrual age (PMA) estimation (in weeks) from brain diffusion MRI of very preterm born infants (born <31weeks gestational age), with an objective to investigate how differences in estimated brain age and PMA were associated with the risk of Cerebral Palsy disorders (CP). Infants were scanned up to 2 times, between 29 and 46 weeks (w) PMA. We applied a deep learning 2D convolutional neural network (CNN) regression model to estimate PMA from local image patches extracted from the diffusion MRI dataset. These were combined to form a global prediction for each MRI scan. We found that CNN can reliably estimate PMA (Pearson's r = 0.6, p < 0.05) from MRIs before 36 weeks of age ('Early' scans). These results revealed that the local fractional anisotropy (FA) measures of these very early scans preserved age specific information. Most interestingly, infants who were later diagnosed with CP were more likely to have an estimated younger brain age from 'Early' scans, the estimated age deviations were significantly different (Regression coefficient: −2.16, p < 0.05, corrected for actual age) compared to those infants who were not diagnosed with CP.

Keywords: Preterm · CNN · Cerebral Palsy · Postmenstrual age
Deep learning

1 Introduction

Infants born very preterm may be at high risk of structural and functional abnormalities of the brain, as well as adverse outcomes including Cerebral Palsy (CP) [1]. Currently, the diagnosis of CP or other motor and cognitive abnormalities are made at approximately 2 years of age [2]. Early detection of developmental abnormalities and thus earlier intervention and treatment are critical to improve outcomes for affected individuals. Brain imaging, such as magnetic resonance imaging (MRI), is one of the techniques to identify early markers of motor or cognitive outcome [3]. Finding an

© Crown 2018
A. Melbourne and R. Licandro et al. (Eds.): DATRA/PIPPI 2018, LNCS 11076, pp. 87–96, 2018.
https://doi.org/10.1007/978-3-030-00807-9_9

early biomarker specific to CP or other types of adverse outcomes is a challenging task [4]. Analyses of large datasets are needed to determine any overlooked and generalized features for early prediction of adverse neurodevelopmental outcome such as CP in preterm infants. For this task, cutting-edge techniques like machine learning or deep learning based technologies may play an important role.

Estimating morphological age and its deviation from the nominal gestational age by atlas based methods from brain MR images has proven useful for assessment of pathologies like lissencephaly [5]. Few studies that used CNN for estimating age (in years) directly from the MRI scans were on adult cohort [6, 7], however, these techniques have not been investigated in preterm infants or for prediction of infants at risk of CP. We propose to use a CNN trained with brain patches to estimate PMA of preterm born infants using brain diffusion MRI. The globally and locally estimated brain ages might be utilized to identify brain structures that indicate of PMA and to determine the correlation of local and global age deviations with clinical phenotype.

Here, we estimated the postmenstrual age (PMA) from diffusion MRI of preterm infants by a deep learning CNN based regression model. Infants were scanned at 2 time points, 'Early' (29.4–35.3 weeks) and 'Term' (age: 38.43–46.6 weeks) PMA. A CNN regression model was trained on a preterm cohort with no evidence of CP at 2 years corrected age, and then tested on the infants with or without a later diagnosis of CP separately. We compared our findings with a brain-volume based age estimation model. Overall, our aim was to investigate whether estimating PMA from MRI of preterm infants is possible in weekly resolution by a patch based CNN model and whether there is any difference in the range of estimated deviations between infants later diagnosed with CP compared to those who were not.

2   Method

2.1   MR Imaging Acquisition

Infants born <31 weeks gestational age (GA) were enrolled and scanned utilizing an MR compatible incubator equipped with a dedicated neonatal head coil (LMT Lammers Medical Technology, Lübeck, Germany) as part of a prospective cohort study [1]. Diffusion images were acquired, consisting of one low (b = 0 s/mm^2) and 64 diffusion-weighted images (2000 s/mm^2), in which the diffusion encoding gradients were uniformly distributed in space. Imaging parameters of the diffusion sequence were: field of view 224×224 mm, matrix 128×128, repetition time 9500 ms, echo time 130 ms and flip angle of 90°. Conventional MRI was conducted to assess brain abnormalities. A total of 119 infants underwent at least the 'Early' MRI. We excluded infants from our study who did not attend follow-up assessment at 2 years, or whose diffusion weighted images were of poor quality. Data of a total of 82 infants not diagnosed with CP (non-CP cohort) and 4 infants diagnosed with CP (CP cohort) at 2 years corrected age were analyzed.

Brain abnormalities were scored using conventional images [8], see Table 1. A histogram on the distribution of age is shown in Fig. 1.

Table 1. MRI based global brain abnormality (according to Kidokoro scores [8]) for the MRIs of preterm infants in our dataset

Classification	Full dataset	Training (non-CP)	Validation (non-CP)	Test (non-CP)	CP
Normal	71	58	8	5	2
Mild abnormality	51	36	6	9	–
Moderate abnormality	13	13	–	–	–
Severe abnormality	6	5	–	1	4
N/A	1	1	–	–	–

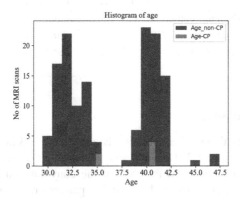

Fig. 1. Distribution of postmenstrual ages at the time of MRI.

2.2 MRI Preprocessing

MRI pre-processing procedures included removal of volumes affected by intra-volume motion, correction of between volume motion including rotation of the b-matrix, correction of image distortions due to susceptibility inhomogeneities using a field map, and detection and replacement of signal intensity outlier slices prior to resampling. Images were upsampled to 1.25 mm isotropic resolution and maps of fractional anisotropy (FA) were estimated using the diffusion tensor model. Brain masks were estimated from the non-diffusion-weighted images using registration to a study specific template and subsequent multi-atlas voting. Brain volumes were calculated from the brain masks. FA images were affinely registered to one of two study specific atlases created separately for the 'Early' and 'Term' time points. The same transformations were applied to the brain masks. All data were normalized to zero mean and unit variance.

2.3   Data Preprocessing for CNN and 'Brain Volume' Model

Our dataset for the non-CP cohort was composed of 142 scans (72 'Early' and 70 'Term' MRI). We used 80% of the scans for training, 10% for validation and 10% for test. Our CP cohort was small with 6 scans (2 'Early' and 4 'Term' MRI) from 4 infants. The same partitions were used for the brain-volume based linear regression model ('Brain Volume' model) for age estimation. For the CNN, 20 × 20 × 20 voxel non-overlapping patches were extracted from the scans within the brain using the brain masks, which were then used to train the network. The number of scans and patches for training, validation and test datasets are listed in Table 2.

Table 2. Number of patches and scans in different datasets used for CNN models

Dataset	No of scans	No of patches
Training (non-CP)	113	7719
Validation (non-CP)	14	898
Test (non-CP)	15	895
CP	6	449

2.4   Network Architecture

The CNN consisted of three 2D convolution layers with 3 × 3 kernel and three max-pooling layers with stride of 2. Dropout was used as regularization to prevent over-fitting. ReLU activation was used for each of the convolutional layers. The final 3 layers were fully connected, which blended the parameters to combine the feature vectors. The output of the network was a scalar, which indicated the predicted brain age for each patch. The learning rate was 0.001 and 'Adam' optimizer was used. The details of this network architecture can be found in Table 3.

Table 3. CNN network architecture

Layer index	Name	Relevant parameters (no of filters, kernel size, number of output neurons, dropout)
1	Conv2D	16@3x3
2	ReLU	N/A
3	Maxpooling 2D	2
4	Dropout	0.8
5	Conv2D	32@3x3
6	ReLU	N/A
7	Maxpooling 2D	2
9	Conv2D	32@3x3
10	ReLU	N/A
11	Maxpooling 2D	2

(*continued*)

Table 3. (*continued*)

Layer index	Name	Relevant parameters (no of filters, kernel size, number of output neurons, dropout)
12	Dropout	0.8
13	Flatten	N/A
14	FC	256
15	Dropout	0.8
16	FC	128
17	Dropout	0.8
18	FC	1
19	Linear	N/A

2.5 Implementation

The CNN was implemented in TensorFlow (1.5.0) on a clustered CPU computation environment. The end-to-end algorithm was written in Python. With CPU computation, the time for training was ~ 2 h and testing was ~ 2 s for each test dataset. For the 'Brain Volume' model, a scikit-learn based linear regression function was used.

2.6 Performance Measures

As a post-processing step (Fig. 2), a single estimated age value was assigned to each scan from the CNN estimation with maximum frequency (mode) over its patches. Pearson correlation coefficients were calculated between actual and predicted PMA for 'Early' and 'Term' patches and scans of 'Validation' and 'Test' datasets. Similarly, correlations were also measured for the 'Brain Volume' model. Bland-Altman plots were generated for analyzing residuals for both of the models. In addition, CNN prediction accuracies for patches and scans at different estimated deviation ranges were reported. Finally, brain age deviation for each scan was calculated from the difference between the model-predicted brain age and actual postmenstrual age for both of the models and compared between non-CP and CP group by histograms, fitted kernel density estimates (KDE) and general linear regression models.

3 Results

We first tested whether our CNN model can estimate the local and global PMA from MRI patches and scans respectively for both preterm infants with and without CP. CNN model predictions for patches for the non-CP 'Validation', non-CP 'Test' and CP scans are shown in Fig. 3A. The Pearson's r between actual and predicted ages was (0.07, p = 0.1) for 'Early' non-CP 'Test' patches and (0.2, p < 0.05) for the 'Term' patches. This poor correlation can be attributed to a high variability in the predicted ages over local patches of any scan. Therefore, after combining the patch-based estimates into a single scan-based estimate (post-processing), r increased to 0.62

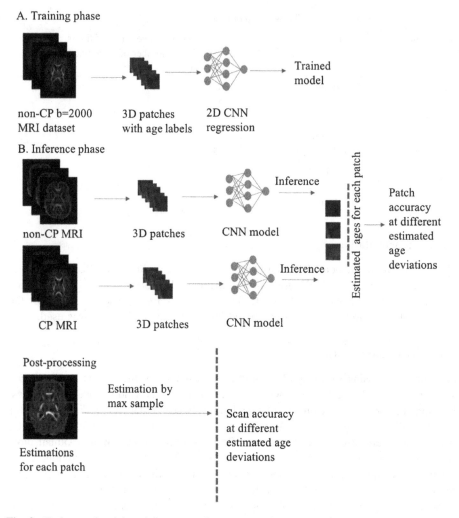

A. Training phase

non-CP b=2000   3D patches   2D CNN
MRI dataset   with age labels   regression

Trained model

B. Inference phase

non-CP MRI   3D patches   CNN model   Inference

CP MRI   3D patches   CNN model   Inference

Estimated ages for each patch

Patch accuracy at different estimated age deviations

Post-processing

Estimation by max sample

Estimations for each patch

Scan accuracy at different estimated age deviations

Fig. 2. End to end training, inference and post-processing phases with a deep learning CNN regression network.

(p = 0.054) for the 'Early' non-CP 'Test' scans and 0.63 (p = 0.25) for 'Term' scans. When the 'Test' and 'Validation' datasets were combined, we found a significant correlation (r = 0.6, p < 0.05) for 'Early' scans and a poor correlation (r = 0.25 p = 0.3) for the 'Term' scans. Thus, despite the variability over local estimations, local patches in scans preserved age specific features in 'Early' MRI. The 'Brain Volume' model predictions also showed a strong correlation for both 'Early' (r = 0.75, p < 0.05) and 'Term' (r = 0.65, p = 0.23) non-CP 'Test' scans. For the combination of 'Validation' and 'Test' scans, r decreased to 0.61 (p < 0.05) for 'Early' scans and to 0.4 (p = 0.22) for 'Term' scans. Thus, both of the models showed a strong age predictability (in weeks) from 'Early' MRI. Predictions from 'Term' MRI were unreliable

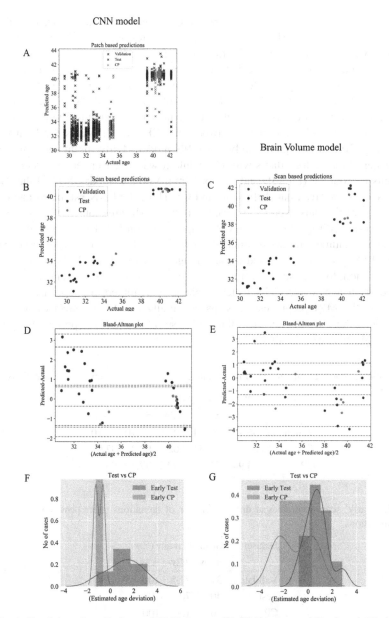

Fig. 3. A. Patch based predictions of PMA in non-CP (Validation and Test) and CP datasets. B and C. Scan based predictions (after post-processing) of PMA in non-CP and CP datasets by CNN and 'Brain Volume' model respectively. D & E: Residual plots for CNN and 'Brain Volume' model, respectively. F & G. Comparison of estimated age deviations between non-CP 'Test' and 'CP' group from CNN and 'Brain Volume' model respectively.

for the CNN model with the particular post-processing scheme and inaccurate for the 'Brain Volume' model as shown by their respective residual plots in Fig. 3D and E. Therefore, we excluded 'Term' predictions from further analysis.

As a secondary analysis, we calculated the patch and scan based prediction accuracy for 'Early' scans only at different age deviations as shown in Tables 4 and 5. The age prediction accuracies for CNN model were 70% for non-CP ('Test') and 100% for CP scans within ±2w deviation. We then compared the distributions in estimated age deviations (for 'Early' scans only) between non-CP and CP scans for both of the models (Fig. 3F and G). Interestingly, for CNN model, 'Early' brain age was consistently underestimated for infants with CP, while it was either under- or overestimated for infants without CP (Fig. 3D and F). For 'Brain Volume' model, 50% of the 'Early' CP scans were underestimated (Fig. 3E and G). Thus, the CNN estimated age deviations for 'Early' scans were significantly reduced (Regression coefficient: -2.16, $p < 0.05$, corrected for actual age) in CP compared to non-CP (Test +Validation) while the 'Brain Volume' model estimated deviations were not (Regression coefficient $= -1.58$, $p = 0.11$, corrected for actual age). For the 'Brain Volume' model, the underestimation for CP scans seems to be related to a smaller brain volume than expected at an age, while CNN features related with underestimation are still to be explored as the MRI preprocessing steps essentially negate the effect of brain size. Nevertheless, these results represent that underestimated brain age preferably by CNN models might indicate risk of CP.

Table 4. Patch accuracies at different ranges of deviations from CNN estimations

Dataset	Patch accuracy (%)				
	±0.5w	±1w	±2w	±3w	±4w
Validation	36.75	58.24	89.75	95.10	95.10
Test	26.03	51.51	86.59	94.30	97.09
CP	73.94	79.51	89.53	97.10	98.89

Table 5. 'Early' scan accuracies at different ranges of deviations (after post processing) from CNN estimations

Dataset	Scan accuracy (%)		
	±1w	±2w	±3w
Validation	37.5	87.5	100
Test	40	70	90
CP	50	100	100

4   Discussion

We presented a CNN based postmenstrual age prediction approach for preterm infants and, to our knowledge, this is the first study to utilize the CNN estimations as a very early predictor of CP. The expected developmental abnormalities of the preterm brain with varying degrees of brain abnormalities made the age prediction task from local brain features challenging. Our study showed that both local brain feature based CNN regression model and total brain volume based linear regression model ('Brain Volume') reliably predicted PMA of the preterm infants from their 'Early' scans with strong correlations and reasonable prediction accuracy within ±2w deviation.

The Bland-Altman plots for CNN predictions (Fig. 3D) appear to show a systematic prediction error (overestimation for younger, underestimation for older) for 'Early' test scans but not for 'Early' validation scans. With only one train/validation/test split, it is difficult to determine whether this is coincidental. Cross-validations are required to verify these findings. More importantly, different types of post processing schemes, which biologically represent how the local age information in the brain is related to a global age, should be explored. Detailed studies on the patches, which are associated with the closest estimation of the actual age, should be conducted and thus only specific regions could be considered while predicting a global age. The brain age prediction was unreliable/inaccurate at term equivalent age for both of the models as indicated by lower Pearson's r correlation and residuals (Fig. 3D and E). The more reliable prediction at younger age could be due to more rapid changes to the brain folding patterns or fractional anisotropy in the early period than later. As a consequence, there may not be enough information in the local features of the 'Term' scans for sufficiently reliable predictions; in addition, the expected abnormal developmental trajectory for the preterm might make the prediction harder. The ideal post-processing scheme might be different between 'Early' and 'Term' scans. In addition, the age band for 'Term' training was fairly narrow.

The most interesting finding is that while the non-CP dataset consisted of some patients with brain abnormality as shown in Table 1, the estimated age deviations from CNN models were significantly different between the 'Early' non-CP and CP groups of scans. The difference was not significant though for 'Brain Volume' model estimations. Nevertheless, the distributions from both of the models as shown in Fig. 3F and G revealed that CP cases are more likely to be underestimated than non-CP ones. In addition, it is noticeable that 100% of the CP scans (Early + Term) in CNN and ∼70% of the CP scans in Brain Volume model were underestimated. This underestimation could be related to smaller brain volumes than normal, and for the CNN, any developmental delay in FA features. A number of previous studies [9, 10] reported the association of head circumference and developmental dysfunction related to CP, while with respect to FA features, previous data [11] showed that children with poor developmental outcomes at the age of 2 have lower FA in specific brain regions. Our study investigated these features at very early stages by utilizing local and global brain age deviations with an aim to find out a distinction line between non-CP and CP scans. It seems that underestimated brain age from the 'Early' scans preferably by CNN model could be one of the diagnostic features of CP, which in combination with other clinical scores could be indicative of CP disorder at a very early stage. Finally, it should be noted that all these observations were made on 2 'Early' and 4 'Term' CP scans and need to be verified on larger cohorts of preterm infants with CP.

One of the main advantages of a patch based CNN approach is that it might be able to identify the local brain patches that contain stronger features for age as well as the patches that show higher estimated deviations and thus could be potentially related to brain abnormalities. Future studies will explore the correlation of CNN model estimations and clinical findings in local brain regions. CNN training with larger samples and with multimodal MRI inputs will likely facilitate this kind of study.

References

1. George, J., et al.: PPREMO: a prospective cohort study of preterm infant brain structure and function to predict neurodevelopmental outcome. BMC Pediatr. **15**(1), 123 (2015)
2. McIntyre, S., Morgan, C., Walker, K., Novak, I.: Cerebral Palsy-don't delay. Dev. Disabil. Res. Rev. **17**(2), 114–129 (2011)
3. George, J., et al.: Relationship between very early brain structure and neuromotor, neurological and neurobehavioral function in infants born <31 weeks gestational age. Early Hum. Dev. **117**, 74–82 (2018)
4. Zhang, J.: Multivariate analysis and machine learning in Cerebral Palsy research. Front. Neurol. **8**, 715 (2017)
5. Dittrich, E., et al.: A spatio-temporal latent atlas for semi-supervised learning of fetal brain segmentations and morphological age estimation. Med. Image Anal. **18**(1), 9–21 (2014)
6. Cole, J., et al.: Predicting brain age with deep learning from raw imaging data results in a reliable and heritable biomarker. NeuroImage **163**, 115–124 (2017)
7. Huang, T., Chen, H., Fujimoto, R.: Age estimation from brain MRI images using deep learning. In: 2017 IEEE 14th International Symposium on Biomedical Imaging (ISBI 2017), Melbourne, VIC, Australia. IEEE (2017)
8. George, J., et al.: Validation of an MRI brain injury and growth scoring system in very preterm infants scanned at 29- to 35-week postmenstrual age. Am. J. Neuroradiol. **38**(7), 1435–1442 (2017)
9. Jensen, A., Holmer, B.: White matter damage in 4,725 term-born infants is determined by head circumference at birth: the missing link. Obstet. Gynecol. Int. **2018**, 1–12 (2018)
10. Kuban, K., et al.: Developmental correlates of head circumference at birth and two years in a cohort of extremely low gestational age newborns. J. Pediatr. **155**(3), 344–349.e3 (2009)
11. Babcock, M., et al.: Injury to the preterm brain and cerebral palsy: clinical aspects, molecular mechanisms, unanswered questions, and future research directions. J. Child Neurol. **24**(9), 1064–1084 (2009)

Segmentation of Pelvic Vessels in Pediatric MRI Using a Patch-Based Deep Learning Approach

A. Virzì[1,4(✉)], P. Gori[1], C. O. Muller[2,4], E. Mille[2,4], Q. Peyrot[2,4], L. Berteloot[3,4], N. Boddaert[3,4], S. Sarnacki[2,4], and I. Bloch[1,4]

[1] LTCI, Télécom ParisTech, Université Paris-Saclay, Paris, France
`alessio.virzi@telecom-paristech.fr`
[2] Department of Pediatric Surgery, Paris Descartes University, Hôpital Necker Enfants-Malades, Assistance Publique - Hôpitaux de Paris, Paris, France
[3] Department of Pediatric Radiology, Paris Descartes University, Hôpital Necker Enfants-Malades, Assistance Publique - Hôpitaux de Paris, Paris, France
[4] IMAG2 Laboratory, Imagine Institute, Paris, France

Abstract. In this paper, we propose a patch-based deep learning approach to segment pelvic vessels in 3D MRI images of pediatric patients. For a given T2 weighted MRI volume, a set of 2D axial patches are extracted using a limited number of user-selected landmarks. In order to take into account the volumetric information, successive 2D axial patches are combined together, producing a set of pseudo RGB color images. These RGB images are then used as input for a convolutional neural network (CNN), pre-trained on the ImageNet dataset, which results into both segmentation and vessel labeling as veins or arteries. The proposed method is evaluated on 35 MRI volumes of pediatric patients, obtaining an average segmentation accuracy in terms of Average Symmetric Surface Distance of $ASSD = 0.89 \pm 0.07\,\mathrm{mm}$ and Dice Index of $DC = 0.79 \pm 0.02$.

1 Introduction

Surgical planning relies on the patient's anatomy and is often based on medical images acquired before the surgery. In particular, this is the case for pelvic surgery where the standard procedure is still to visually analyze, slice by slice, the images of the pelvic region. This operation can be quite difficult and tedious due to the complexity and variability of the pelvic structures. Furthermore, it is even more complicated in the case of children, since the anatomy varies over time and it is specific to the age of the patient. Difficulties are emphasized when dealing with pathological cases such as malformations or tumors. For these reasons, it is very important and challenging, especially for children, to provide surgeons with patient-specific 3D models, obtained from the segmentation of anatomical images.

© Springer Nature Switzerland AG 2018
A. Melbourne and R. Licandro et al. (Eds.): DATRA/PIPPI 2018, LNCS 11076, pp. 97–106, 2018.
https://doi.org/10.1007/978-3-030-00807-9_10

In this paper, we propose a method to segment the pelvic vessels. Within all pelvic structures, vessels are particularly important since they need to be preserved during surgery in order to avoid potential functional damages to the patient's organs.

Most of the studies on vessels segmentation are dedicated to adult patients and applied to contrast-enhanced imaging modalities, such as computed tomography angiography (CTA) or magnetic resonance angiography (MRA) images, as extensively described in [1,2]. These image modalities often rely on the injection of a contrast agent and on specific acquisition protocols, producing vessels-enhanced images.

However, the use of contrast agents is not always recommended in clinical practice, especially for pediatric patients [3]. For this reason, standard MRI acquisitions are usually chosen for pediatric pelvis exams. The choice of MRI, instead of other modalities such as CT, is also related to its non-irradiating nature, which is very important in pediatrics, and to its good contrast resolution of the soft tissues [4,5]. The use of standard MRI makes it difficult to apply the methods developed for angiography images, since they are specifically designed for strong vessels enhanced images. Moreover, for pediatric patients, there are harder clinical constraints on the scan acquisition time than for adults, which do not allow to considerably increase the images resolution. This, coupled with a smaller size of the vessels walls for pediatric patients, produces images with higher partial volume effects compared to adults. These partial volume effects could locally create weak or missing boundaries, which makes it even more difficult to apply classical methods such as level-sets [6]. This shows why there is a need for segmentation methods specifically conceived for pediatric imaging.

In the last years, deep learning methods and in particular convolutional neural networks (CNNs) have shown excellent performances in various medical imaging tasks [7]. However, deep learning methods usually require a huge number of manually annotated data, which is really difficult to obtain in the medical field, and especially in pediatrics. To this end, recent studies [8–11] have relied on transfer learning [12] from pre-trained networks on large datasets of natural images (e.g. ImageNet [13]). However, these studies cannot be directly applied to volumetric data, due to the nature of the training dataset (e.g. 2D color images for ImageNet). Moreover, discarding the 3D nature of medical images would result in a loss of useful information for the segmentation task. For this reason, some studies [10,11] successfully proposed to generate 2D pseudo-color images from volumetric gray-level images, aiming to incorporate 3D information.

In this paper, we propose a patch-based deep learning approach that is, to the best of our knowledge, the first study on pelvic vessels segmentation with pediatric MRI. Starting from a set of user-selected landmarks, a series of patches containing the structures of interest is extracted. In this way, for each patient, the user can focus on the analysis of the vascular structures of surgical interest. Similarly to [11], the patches are generated by stacking the gray levels information of successive slices (Sect. 2.1), forming pseudo-RGB images.

This approach allows us to take into account the 3D information of the image while using a CNN pre-trained on ImageNet (Sect. 2.2).

2   Vessels Segmentation and Labeling

The proposed method for the segmentation of the pelvic vessels consists of two main steps: a semi-automatic extraction of a set of axial patches containing the vascular structures of interest, followed by an automatic segmentation procedure based on CNN and transfer learning. The pipeline of the proposed method is depicted in Fig. 1.

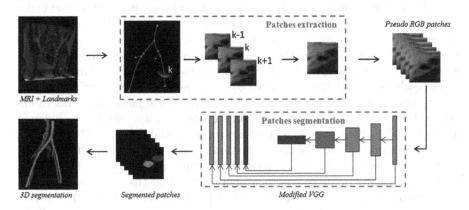

Fig. 1. Pipeline of the proposed method. A set of 2D pseudo-RGB patches are extracted from the MRI volume and from a set of user-selected landmarks. Patches are then segmented through a modified version [11] of the VGG network [14], obtaining the 3D segmentation of the vessels.

Preprocessing. First, histogram equalization of each MRI volume is performed. Then, in order to reduce the noise, an anisotropic diffusion filter [15] is applied, taking into account the tubular structure of the vessels.

2.1   Patches Extraction

The definition of patches relies on three steps. First, some landmarks along the vessels are provided by the user. The only constraint is that these points should belong to the vessels. In particular, in case of bifurcations, the user can select landmarks on vessel branches in any order. The other two steps, detailed next, consist in reconstructing the vascular tree from the landmarks, and in defining patches centered on the vessels branches in each slice of the image volume.

Vascular Tree Reconstruction. Let $L = \{\varphi_i = (x_i, y_i, z_i) \in \Omega, i \in \{1...n\}\}$ be the set of user-selected landmarks, where $n = |L|$ is the number of landmarks, $\Omega \subseteq \mathbb{R}^3$ is the image domain, and L is ordered decreasingly in z ($\forall i \in \{1...n-1\}, z_{i+1} \leq z_i$), hence in the cranio-caudal direction. The vascular tree is reconstructed iteratively by choosing, at each step i, the best candidate landmark $\varphi_c = (x_c, y_c, z_c)$ to be connected with φ_i, minimizing the following objective function, which combines shape and appearance information:

$$f(\varphi_i, \varphi_c) = \alpha||\varphi_i - \varphi_c||_2 + \beta\kappa(\varphi_i, \varphi_c, \varphi_{c-1}) + \gamma\sigma^2_{(\varphi_i, \varphi_c)} \,,$$

where φ_{c-1} is the landmark already connected with φ_c, such that $z_{c-1} > z_c$, κ is the local curvature, estimated as $\frac{1}{r}$ where r is the radius of the circle passing through the three points, σ^2 is the variance of the image intensity in a cylinder whose axis is the line joining φ_i and φ_c and whose circular basis has a fixed radius r_c, and α, β, γ are constant weight values. Minimizing f means that the path should be formed by points as close as possible, forming a line as straight as possible, and whose spatial context is homogeneous in terms of intensity.

For each iteration i, the candidates φ_c are chosen as the landmarks that have $z_c > z_i$ and that are already connected to at most one landmark. This candidates selection allows us to take into account that, in the pelvis, the different vessels branches are descending along the cranio-caudal direction. Furthermore, we can also automatically handle bifurcation points while avoiding anatomically incoherent connection (i.e. trifurcations). This procedure, repeated for each φ_i, results in an approximate reconstruction of the vascular tree, as shown in Fig. 2. The parameters for the reconstruction are experimentally set to $\alpha = 1$, $\beta = 200$, $\gamma = 10^3$, $r_c = 1$ mm, producing a correct vascular tree reconstruction for all the patients present in the dataset.

Pseudo-RGB Patch Extraction. Once the vascular tree is obtained, each vessel branch is approximated by a spline. For every slice k, we first define p_k as the point where the spline intersects slice k. Then we extract a square patch ($N \times N$ pixels) centered at p_k. Every triple of successive patches ($k - 1$, k and $k + 1$) is interpreted as a pseudo-RGB patch, that incorporates the 3D information of successive patches. This procedure produces a set of pseudo-RGB patches, containing the vascular structures, that will be used as input for the segmentation method that follows.

2.2 Deep CNN for Patches Segmentation

In this section, we propose to use CNN to segment the patches into vessel and non-vessel regions, and jointly classify the vessel regions into veins or arteries. To this aim, a modified version of the VGG-16 network [14], pre-trained on the ImageNet dataset [13] is employed.

The network is built by removing the final fully connected layers of the pre-trained VGG-16 network, while preserving the 5 convolutional stages which constitute the *base network*. Each of these stages consists of Convolutional layers

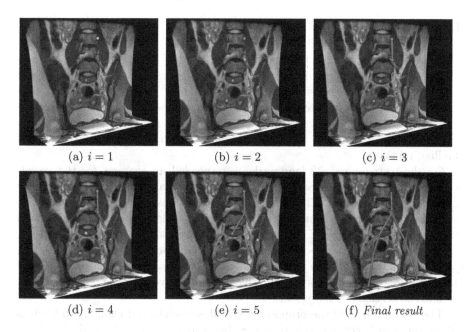

(a) $i = 1$ (b) $i = 2$ (c) $i = 3$

(d) $i = 4$ (e) $i = 5$ (f) *Final result*

Fig. 2. Example of reconstruction of the vascular tree (fist five steps). In each image each blue sphere is a generic landmark, the yellow sphere is the landmark φ_i analyzed at step i and the green spheres are the candidate landmarks for connection φ_c. The vessel paths are represented in red. (Color figure online)

and Rectified Linear Unit layers. Each convolutional stage is connected with the following one by a Max Pooling layer. Starting from this *base network*, a modified network is then added, similarly to [9,11], where a specialized convolutional layer (3×3 kernel size) with 16 features maps is inserted after the last convolutional layer of each stage. These specialized layers are resized to the original image size and concatenated together. Finally, the feature maps in the concatenated layers are linearly combined through a final convolutional layer (1×1 kernel), in order to produce the output segmented image.

As previously mentioned, the layers of the *base network* are already pre-trained on the large ImageNet dataset of natural RGB images. For our application, the entire network is then fine-tuned with a training set of manually segmented patches. Each annotated patch consists of three labels, corresponding to vein, artery and background pixels. The network is trained for 115 k iterations, with a constant learning rate $lr = 10^{-6}$, using a multinomial logistic loss function. The loss function is minimized using a stochastic gradient descent with momentum $m = 0.95$.

The analyzed patches, obtained as described in Sect. 2.1 and segmented using the CNN previously described, are then restored to their original position in the image domain $\Omega \in \mathbb{R}^3$, thus providing a classification into veins, artery and background of the whole image volume.

3 Results

The image dataset used in this study is composed of 35 T2 weighted MRI volumes, of patients between 1 and 18 years old. Images have different sizes and resolutions (average voxel size $0.92 \times 0.92 \times 0.74\,\text{mm}^3$).

All pelvic vessels of interest were manually segmented by medical experts and labeled as veins or arteries. In particular, the following structures were segmented: the abdominal aorta, the inferior vena cava, the iliac arteries and the iliac veins.

On the tested cases, 12 landmarks were needed, in average, for the vessels paths reconstruction (see Sect. 2.1), which required an interaction time of few minutes for each patient. The only guideline for the user was to select the landmarks inside the vessels lumen, which is easier to achieve by navigating through the axial views. This type of interaction was found reasonable by medical experts, and was considered as a good guarantee to obtain good results from the subsequent automatic steps. The patches dimensions were set to 31×31 pixels. Given the resolution of the images and the thickness of the vessels, the patches largely include the sections of the vessels.

The performance of the proposed method was evaluated using a 5-fold cross validation, which corresponds to a training and test set of 28 and 7 patients for each fold respectively. The segmentation accuracy was evaluated in terms of Average Symmetric Surface Distance (ASSD [mm]) and Dice Index (DC) between the proposed segmentation A and the corresponding manual segmentation B provided by a medical expert:

$$DC(A, B) = \frac{2|A \cap B|}{|A| + |B|},$$

$$ASSD = \frac{1}{|S(A)| + |S(B)|} \left(\sum_{s_A \in S(A)} \min_{s_B \in S(B)} \|s_A - s_B\|_2 + \sum_{s_B \in S(B)} \min_{s_A \in S(A)} \|s_A - s_B\|_2 \right),$$

where $S(A)$ and $S(B)$ are the sets of surface voxels of A and B, s_A and s_B are points on $S(A)$ and $S(B)$ respectively. For each patient, these measures were evaluated for both the global vascular segmentation (fusion of vein and artery) and for veins and arteries separately. The average quantitative results for each fold are reported in Table 1.

The results in terms of ASSD, taking into account the images resolution, were considered satisfying by medical experts for surgical planning applications. As expected, results for a single structure (i.e. either artery or vein) were less accurate compared to the overall segmentation. This is mostly due to the additional classification task challenge. Nevertheless, the limited differences between the Dice indices of the three columns in Table 1 indicate an overall good classification performance.

Table 1. Quantitative evaluation of the segmentation results.

	Arteries		Veins		Arteries & Veins	
	DC	ASSD	DC	ASSD	DC	ASSD
Fold 1	0.77	1.45	0.78	1.04	0.80	0.88
Fold 2	0.71	1.38	0.72	2.21	0.79	0.96
Fold 3	0.74	1.33	0.72	1.42	0.78	0.84
Fold 4	0.74	1.31	0.78	1.46	0.81	0.80
Fold 5	0.71	1.58	0.72	1.30	0.76	0.95
Mean ± std	0.73 ± 0.02	1.41 ± 0.11	0.75 ± 0.03	1.49 ± 0.44	0.79 ± 0.02	0.89 ± 0.07

Some qualitative results are shown in Fig. 3. In order to correctly interpret them, it is important to consider the anatomy of the vascular structures. The veins, due to their non rigid internal musculature, tend to collapse more than the arteries. This behavior usually leads to arteries that have a more circular shape in the axial section than veins. As shown in Fig. 3(a) and (b), this feature appears to be effectively incorporated in our method, providing an overall good veins/arteries classification. Furthermore, we also noticed that most of the mis-classification cases were locally confined to regions where this "shape feature" was not expressed. An illustrative example is shown in Fig. 3(c), where a vein with a strong circular shape is erroneously labeled as artery by our method. However, as can be seen in the 3D model of Fig. 3(d), the overall classification is very satisfying and was positively evaluated by medical experts.

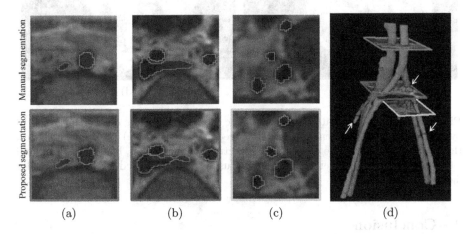

(a)   (b)   (c)   (d)

Fig. 3. Examples of segmentation results. In (a), (b) and (c) the results on some axial sections are depicted. The red contours correspond to the arteries, and the blue ones to the veins. The final 3D model obtained from the segmentation is depicted in (d) with the same color conventions. The three patches in (a), (b) and (c) are shown in (d) with three different colors. Some examples of misclassification are indicated by white arrows. (Color figure online)

Another qualitative result is shown in Fig. 4. It depicts the clinical relevance of the pelvic vessels segmentation in a pediatric patient (8 years old) affected by ovarian teratoma. As it is possible to see, the patient-specific 3D model eases the analysis of the spatial relations between the tumor and the right iliac vessels, which is essential for surgical planning.

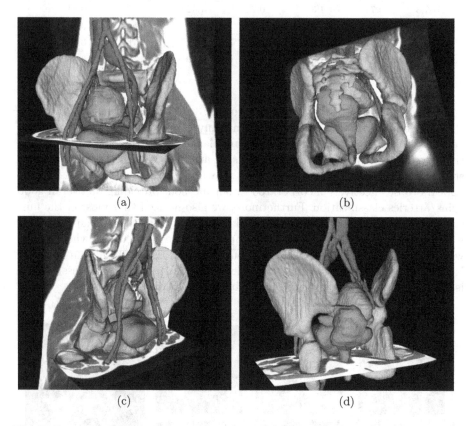

(a)   (b)

(c)   (d)

Fig. 4. Example of 3D patient-specific pelvic model of a 8 years old patient, affected by ovarian teratoma (green). The arteries (red) and veins (blue) are segmented with the proposed method. The other pelvic structures (bones, colon, bladder, sacrum and left ovary) are segmented either manually or using other dedicated methods [4]. (Color figure online)

4   Conclusion

In this paper we presented, to the best of our knowledge, the first study on pelvic vessels segmentation of pediatric MRI. We proposed a patch-based deep learning approach using transfer learning.

A main contribution of this paper was the design of a semi-automatic method for the patches extraction, based on the structural information of the pelvic vascular tree. This approach allows the user to focus, for each patient, on the vascular structures of surgical interest, while avoiding potential unexpected results. We also propose to use pseudo-RGB color patches, that incorporate the 3D information of successive slices. The use of these patches makes it possible to exploit a 2D CNN pre-trained on the ImageNet dataset, which drastically decreases the number of images needed for training. This is fundamental for medical applications where the number of annotated images is limited. It is important to remark that the same strategy, based on transfer learning, would have been difficult to employ with 3D CNNs. In fact, even if efficient implementations of 3D CNNs have been released [16], there is a lack of publicly available 3D CNN models pre-trained on large datasets of 3D images.

As future work, we plan to post-process our results in order to improve the vein/artery classification. This could be done by analyzing the spatial consistency of the classes along the entire 3D model. Moreover, we also plan to investigate other methodologies that take into account the 3D information using more than three successive slices.

Finally, we plan to integrate this method into a complete framework for surgical planning, that will include the semi-automatic segmentation and the 3D visualization of the entire pelvic region (i.e. vessels, nerve fibers, bones ...), using the 3D Slicer software [17]. This will thus provide the surgeon with a complete 3D digital model of the patient (see Fig. 4).

Acknowledgements. A. Virzì, P. Gori, C.O. Muller, E. Mille, Q. Peyrot, L. Berteloot, N. Boddaert, S. Sarnacki and I. Bloch have no conflicts of interest or financial ties to disclose.

References

1. Kirbas, C., Quek, F.: A review of vessel extraction techniques and algorithms. ACM Comput. Surv. (CSUR) **36**(2), 81–121 (2004)
2. Lesage, D., Angelini, E.D., Bloch, I., Funka-Lea, G.: A review of 3D vessel lumen segmentation techniques: models, features and extraction schemes. Med. Image Anal. **13**(6), 819–845 (2009)
3. Sundgren, P.C., Leander, P.: Is administration of gadoliniumbased contrast media to pregnant women and small children justified? J. Magn. Reson. Imaging **34**(4), 750–757 (2011)
4. Virzí, A., et al.: A new method based on template registration and deformable models for pelvic bones semi-automatic segmentation in pediatric MRI. In: IEEE 14th International Symposium on Biomedical Imaging (ISBI), pp. 323–326 (2017)
5. Muller, C., et al.: Towards building 3D individual models from MRI segmentation and tractography to enhance surgical planning for pediatric pelvic tumors and malformations. In: Surgetica, Strasbourg, France, pp. 113–115 (2017)
6. Angelini, E., Jin, Y., Laine, A.: State of the art of level set methods in segmentation and registration of medical imaging modalities. In: Handbook of Biomedical Image Analysis - Registration Models, pp. 47–102. Kluwer Academic/Plenum Publishers, Springer (2005)

7. Litjens, G., et al.: A survey on deep learning in medical image analysis. Med. Image Anal. **42**, 60–88 (2017)
8. Bar, Y., Diamant, I., Wolf, L., Lieberman, S., Konen, E., Greenspan, H.: Chest pathology detection using deep learning with non-medical training. In: IEEE 12th International Symposium on Biomedical Imaging (ISBI), pp. 294–297 (2015)
9. Maninis, K.-K., Pont-Tuset, J., Arbeláez, P., Van Gool, L.: Deep retinal image understanding. In: Ourselin, S., Joskowicz, L., Sabuncu, M.R., Unal, G., Wells, W. (eds.) MICCAI 2016. LNCS, vol. 9901, pp. 140–148. Springer, Cham (2016). https://doi.org/10.1007/978-3-319-46723-8_17
10. Shin, H.C., et al.: Deep convolutional neural networks for computer-aided detection: CNN architectures, dataset characteristics and transfer learning. IEEE Trans. Med. Imaging **35**(5), 1285–1298 (2016)
11. Xu, Y., Géraud, T., Bloch, I.: From neonatal to adult brain MR image segmentation in a few seconds using 3D-like fully convolutional network and transfer learning. In: 23rd IEEE International Conference on Image Processing (ICIP), pp. 4417–4421, Beijing, China (2017)
12. Pan, S.J., Yang, Q.: A survey on transfer learning. IEEE Trans. Knowl. Data Eng. **22**(10), 1345–1359 (2010)
13. Deng, J., Dong, W., Socher, R., Li, L.J., Li, K., Fei-Fei, L.: ImageNet: a large-scale hierarchical image database. In: IEEE Conference on Computer Vision and Pattern Recognition (CVPR) (2009)
14. Simonyan, K., Zisserman, A.: Very deep convolutional networks for large-scale image recognition. CoRR abs/1409.1556 (2014)
15. Perona, P., Malik, J.: Scale-space and edge detection using anisotropic diffusion. IEEE Trans. Pattern Anal. Mach. Intell. **12**(7), 629–639 (1990)
16. Kamnitsas, K., et al.: Efficient multi-scale 3D CNN with fully connected CRF for accurate brain lesion segmentation. Med. Image Anal. **36**, 61–78 (2017)
17. Fedorov, A., et al.: 3D slicer as an image computing platform for the quantitative imaging network. Magn. Reson. Imaging **30**(9), 1323–1341 (2012)

Multi-view Image Reconstruction: Application to Fetal Ultrasound Compounding

Veronika A. Zimmer$^{(\boxtimes)}$, Alberto Gomez, Yohan Noh, Nicolas Toussaint, Bishesh Khanal, Robert Wright, Laura Peralta, Milou van Poppel, Emily Skelton, Jacqueline Matthew, and Julia A. Schnabel

School of Biomedical Engineering and Imaging Sciences, King's College London, London, UK
veronika.zimmer@kcl.ac.uk

Abstract. Ultrasound (US), a standard diagnostic tool to detect fetal abnormalities, is a direction dependent imaging modality, i.e. the position of the probe highly influences the appearance of the image. View-dependent artifacts such as shadows can obstruct parts of the anatomy of interest and degrade the quality and usefulness of the image. If multiple images of the same structure are acquired from different views, view-dependent artifacts can be minimized.

In this work, we propose a new US image reconstruction technique using multiple B-spline grids to enable multi-view US image compounding. The B-spline coefficients of different control point grids adapted to the geometry of the data are simultaneously optimized at every resolution level. Data points are weighted depending on their view, position and intensity. We demonstrate our method on the compounding of co-planar 2D fetal US images acquired from multiple views. Using quantitative and qualitative evaluation scores, we show that the proposed method outperforms other multi-view compounding methods.

1 Introduction

Ultrasound (US) is an imaging technique using high-frequency sound waves to visualize soft tissues and organs inside the body. US is used as a routine diagnostic tool to detect fetal abnormalities. The diagnostic value of US images is limited by the expertise of the operator and the image quality. View-dependent artifacts such as shadows can obstruct parts of the anatomy of interest and degrade the quality and usefulness of the image.

The position of the probe highly influences the appearance of the image. Focal depth is typically set such that the center of the image achieves higher quality. Some of the most degrading artifacts are acoustic shadows (Fig. 1(a)/(b)), which obscure regions of the image, and changes in pixel intensity with depth due to tissue attenuation, which cannot always be compensated for using time gain

© Springer Nature Switzerland AG 2018
A. Melbourne and R. Licandro et al. (Eds.): DATRA/PIPPI 2018, LNCS 11076, pp. 107–116, 2018.
https://doi.org/10.1007/978-3-030-00807-9_11

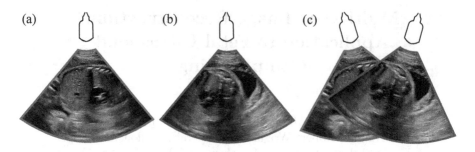

Fig. 1. (a)/(b) US images from different view directions with shadow artifacts; (c) co-planar alignment of both views, which are acquired with two active transducers.

compensation (TGC) accurately. If multiple images of the same structure are acquired from different views, view-dependent artifacts can be minimized. This can yield an easier and improved delineation of the detailed fetal anatomy by the sonographers.

Previous work has focused on compounding of multi-view 3D volumes, where there is some overlap of the fields of view (FoV) [1–3]. However, 2D imaging provides better image quality and higher frame rate and is the main imaging mode in fetal screening protocols. But obtaining a coincident imaging plane for multi-view compounding with a freehand 2D transducer is nearly impossible in practice.

In this work, we focus on the compounding of fetal 2D multi-view US images. To this end, we use a custom-made modification to a standard ultrasound system to connect two active transducers, and a physical device to maintain them on the same imaging plane, see Fig. 1(c).

To compound the multi-view images, we propose a new B-spline based [4] image reconstruction method. Due to the lack of a ground truth, different compounding methods were compared and rated qualitatively by experts, indicating a higher image quality when using multiple polar grids and a data point weighting.

Our main contributions are three-fold. First, we define multiple, view-dependent B-spline grids, adapted to the intrinsic polar geometry of US images. The US signal is measured in a polar coordinate system and only afterwards scan converted to Cartesian coordinates and interpolated for visualization. To obtain a single multi-view image, the B-spline coefficients of the grids are then determined simultaneously. Second, we introduce a data point weighting in the B-spline formulation based on the position (not only on the beam angles as in [5]) and on the intensities. And third, we evaluate our method on a dataset of 2D fetal US images acquired from multiple co-planar views.

2   Methods

2.1   Classical B-Spline Approximation

Let $\mathbf{X} = \{\mathbf{x}_n\}_{n=1}^N \in \Omega \subset \mathbb{R}^2$ with $\mathbf{x}_n = (x_n, y_n)$ be a set of N image sampling points and $\mathbf{f} = f_n \in \mathbb{R}$ corresponding image intensities. The aim is to find a function $\mathcal{S}(\mathbf{x})$ such that $\mathcal{S}(\mathbf{x}_n) \approx f_n$. Using B-splines, this function can be expressed as

$$\mathcal{S}(\mathbf{x}; \mathbf{w}) = \sum_{p,q} \beta(\frac{x}{a} - p)\beta(\frac{y}{b} - q)w_{p,q},$$

where p, q are the indices of the grid control points, $w_{p,q}$ their coefficients, a, b the grid spacings along x- and y-direction with grid size $N^p \times N^q$, and $\beta(\cdot)$ is the B-spline basis function of degree d. Now, one has to find the coefficient vector $\mathbf{w}^* = (w_{p,q})$ such that

$$\mathbf{w}^* = \underset{\mathbf{w}}{\operatorname{argmin}} \sum_n \| \mathcal{S}(\mathbf{x}_n; \mathbf{w}) - f_n \|^2 + \lambda R(\mathcal{S}(\mathbf{x}; \mathbf{w})),$$

where $\mathcal{R}$ is a regularization term and $\lambda \in \mathbb{R}$ a weighting parameter accounting for the trade-off between the reconstruction accuracy and the smoothness of the function $\mathcal{S}$.

For each point $\mathbf{x}_n$, the B-spline expansion $\mathcal{S}$ can be expressed in matrix form as $\mathcal{S}(\mathbf{x}_n) = B_n\mathbf{w}$ with $B_n = [b_{0,0}(\mathbf{x}_n)\ b_{0,1}(\mathbf{x}_n)\dots b_{N^p,N^q}(\mathbf{x}_n)] \in \mathbb{R}^{N^p \cdot N^q}$ and $b_{p,q} = \beta(\frac{x}{a} - p)\beta(\frac{y}{b} - q)$. For all image points, this can be written as $\mathbf{f} = B\mathbf{w}$, where the nth row of $B \in \mathbb{R}^{N \times (N^p \cdot N^q)}$ is B_n, corresponding to image point $\mathbf{x}_n$. The coefficient vector $\mathbf{w}^*$ is then calculated by [6]

$$\mathbf{w}^* = (B^T B + \lambda R)^{-1} B^T \mathbf{f}. \tag{1}$$

A widely used strategy, adopted in this work, is to compute the B-spline expansion on multiple resolution levels $l = 0, \dots, L$ [4]. On the coarsest level $l = 0$, the function $\mathcal{S}_l$ is approximating the image intensities $\mathbf{f}$. On all subsequent levels $l > 0$, $\mathcal{S}_l(\mathbf{x}_n)$ is fitted against the residual $r_n = \mathbf{f}_n - (\sum_{l=1}^L \mathcal{S}_l(\mathbf{x}_n))$. The coefficients for each level are summed up for the final B-spline reconstruction.

2.2   Data Point Weighting Scheme

The contribution of each image point n can be weighted by a scalar $c_n \in \mathbb{R}^+$, $\sum_n c_n = N$. By arranging these weights in the diagonal of a weight matrix $C \in \mathbb{R}^{N^p \cdot N^q} \times \mathbb{R}^{N^p \cdot N^q}$, the weights can be incorporated into Eq. (1) as

$$\mathbf{w}^* = (B^T C B + \lambda R)^{-1} B^T C \mathbf{f}. \tag{2}$$

Our proposed weighting scheme is motivated by the widely used maximum compounding technique, where for the fusion of two images always the pixel value with maximum intensity is selected. Therefore, the weights in Eq. (2) are chosen such that data points with a strong signal have higher weights: $c_n = \frac{N}{\sum_i^N f_i} f_n$.

Additionally, we propose to take into account the position of a data point in the image. At acquisition time, image settings are optimized to get the best quality in the center, where the object of interest will be. We formulate the weight of data point $\mathbf{x}_n$ as a function of the depth with respect to the probe position $\mathbf{b} \in \mathbb{R}^2$ and the beam angle $\alpha_n \in \mathbb{R}$:

$$g_n = g(\mathbf{x}_n, \alpha_n, \mathbf{b}) = \frac{1}{2\pi} \exp\left(-\left(\frac{\| \mathbf{x}_n - \mathbf{b} \|^2}{2\sigma_1^2} + \frac{\alpha_n}{2\sigma_2^2}\right)\right)$$

$$c_n = \frac{N}{\sum_i^N g_i f_i} g_n f_n \tag{3}$$

with standard deviations $\sigma_1, \sigma_2 \in \mathbb{R}$. Using the Gaussian kernel $g(\mathbf{x}_n, \alpha_n, \mathbf{b})$, a higher weight is given to data points closer to the transducer and with small beam angles. σ_1 and σ_2 were chosen to get high weights at the center of the image.

2.3   Multi-view Image Reconstruction

The matrix formulation of the B-spline approximation problem is convenient for the incorporation of multiple grids of different geometry.

Particularly, we propose to use multiple polar B-spline grids, which are adapted to the US acquisition geometry. Single polar grids have been used before for example for cardiac US registration [7]. Polar coordinates (r, θ) can be parameterized as $\mathbf{x} \in \mathbb{R}^2, \mathbf{x} = (x, y)^T$: $x = r\sin(\theta)$ and $y = r\cos(\theta)$.

US images from different views do not share the same polar coordinate system. To account for this, we propose to use a separate grid for each view (as illustrated in Fig. 2(b)/(c) for two views) and optimize the coefficients of all grids simultaneously at each resolution level.

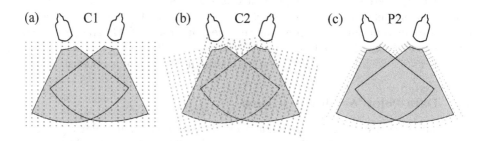

Fig. 2. Geometry of control point grids. (a) C1, single uniform (Cartesian) grid; (b) C2, two uniform (Cartesian) grids; (c) P2, two polar grids.

We consider T US views of the same object, acquired from different directions. The spatial transformations $\phi_t : \mathbb{R}^2 \to \mathbb{R}^2$, $t = 1, \ldots, T$, align the T views. Those transformations can be obtained for example using image registration, tracker information or are known a priori due to special system settings.

At resolution level l, we construct T B-spline matrices $B_t, t = 1, \ldots, T$, with $B_t = [b_{0,0}(\phi_t(\mathbf{x}_n))\ b_{0,1}(\phi_t(\mathbf{x}_n)) \ldots b_{N_t^p, N_t^q}(\phi_t(\mathbf{x}_n))] \in \mathbb{R}^{N_t}$. Here, $N_t = N_t^p \cdot N_t^q$ is the number of control points for view t with grid size $N_t^p \times N_t^q$. For each view, a separate coefficient vector $\mathbf{w}_t \in \mathbb{R}^{N_t}$ has to be calculated. This is done by concatenating the B_t's to a single matrix $B \in \mathbb{R}^{N \times (N_1 + N_2 + \cdots + N_T)}$ as $B = [B_1\ B_2 \cdots B_T]$.

With the regularization matrix $R \in \mathbb{R}^{(N_1 + N_2 + \cdots + N_T) \times (N_1 + N_2 + \cdots + N_T)}$

$$
R = \begin{pmatrix} R_1 & 0 & \ldots & 0 \\ 0 & R_2 & & \\ & & \ddots & 0 \\ 0 & & 0 & R_T \end{pmatrix},
$$

Equation (1) is solved and the coefficient vectors $\mathbf{w}_t$ are optimized simultaneously.

3 Materials and Experiments

3.1 Data Acquisition

We use a custom-made US signal multiplexer which allows to connect multiple US transducers to a standard US system, and switches rapidly between them so that images from each transducer are acquired alternatively. If the frame rate is high (as is generally in 2D mode, typically $> 20\,\mathrm{Hz}$), the images from both transducers are acquired nearly at the same time. We use a physical device that keeps the transducers' imaging planes co-planar and that ensures a large overlap in the center of the images to capture the region of interest from two different view angles (see Figs. 1 and 2). The relative position of the images is constant and known by calibration. If fetal motion occurred during the alternating transducer switch, images were discarded. 25 image pairs from five patients (gestational age 20–30w) were acquired using a Philips EPIQ 7g and two x6-1 transducers in 2D mode.

US images are acquired in polar coordinates. As a post-processing step, the recorded US signals are scan converted to a Cartesian coordinate system and spatially interpolated to form a 2D image. We use the scan converted but not interpolated data as input to our method to reduce interpolation artifacts.

3.2 Experiments

B-Spline Fitting Using Data Geometry. We evaluated the effect of using control point grids of different geometry for B-spline fitting of single views (Cartesian vs. polar). For a fair comparison, we ensured that the spacing of the grid points is similar in the center of the image. The grid spacing of the last and finest resolution level was $0.89 \times 1.23\,\mathrm{mm}$ for the Cartesian grid and for the polar grid $0.89 \times 0.22\,\mathrm{mm}$ (close to the probe), $0.89 \times 1.01\,\mathrm{mm}$ (center of image) and $0.89 \times 1.77\,\mathrm{mm}$ (furthest to the transducer).

Multi-view Image Compounding. We compared different multi-view B-spline reconstructions. The methods differ in the number of control point grids, T (see Sect. 2.3), the geometry of the grids and the data point weighting. We compared the following grid (compare Fig. 2) and weighting configurations:

- C1: A single uniform (Cartesian) grid of control points (Fig. 2(a)).
- C2: Two uniform (Cartesian) grids of control points transformed rigidly according to the alignment of the two views (Fig. 2(b)).
- P2: Two polar grids of control points transformed rigidly according to the alignment of the two views (Fig. 2(c)).
- W0: No data point weighting.
- W1: Data point weighting according to Eq. (3).

Accordingly, the method C1W0 denotes a B-spline fitting with a single Cartesian grid and without data point weighting. In total, six methods are compared.

3.3   Evaluation

Quantitative Evaluation. We selected four complementary quality measures to compare reconstructions I to a reference image J (available only for the first experiment): the Mean Square Error (MSE, compares the intensities of two images), the Peak Signal to Noise Ratio (PSNR, accesses the noise level of an image w.r.t. a reference image), the Structural Similarity Index (SSIM, compares structural information, such as luminance and contrast [8]), and the Variance of the Laplacian (VarL, estimates the amount of blur in an image [9]). Given two images $I, J \in \mathbb{R}^{M_1 \times M_2}$, the measures MSE, PSNR, SSIM and VarL are defined as:

$$\text{MSE}(I, J) = \frac{1}{M_1 M_2} \sum_{i=1}^{M_1} \sum_{j=1}^{M_2} (I(i,j) - J(i,j))^2,$$

$$\text{PSNR}(I, J) = 10 \log_{10} \left(\frac{\max(I)}{\text{MSE}(I, J)} \right),$$

$$\text{SSIM}(I, J) = \frac{(2\mu_I \mu_J + c_1)(2\sigma_{IJ} + c_2)}{(\mu_I^2 + \mu_J^2 + c_1)(\sigma_I^2 + \sigma_J^2 + c_2)},$$

$$\text{VarL}(I) = \sum_{i=1}^{M_1} \sum_{j=1}^{M_2} (|L(i,j)| - \bar{L})^2,$$

where $\mu_I, \mu_J, \sigma_I, \sigma_J, \sigma_{IJ} \in \mathbb{R}$ are the means, standard deviation and cross-covariance for images I, J, $c_1, c_2 \in \mathbb{R}$ small constants close to zero, $L \in \mathbb{R}^{M_1 \times M_2}$ the Laplacian image of I and $\bar{L} = \frac{1}{M_1 M_2} \sum_{i=1}^{M_1} \sum_{j=1}^{M_2} |L(i,j)|$.

Qualitative Evaluation. No ground truth is available for the compounding of multiple views and only VarL scores can be computed. Therefore, we additionally designed a qualitative evaluation strategy. We asked seven experts (three clinical and four US engineering experts) to evaluate as follows: at a time, two compounded images obtained by different methods from the same image pair are presented to the rater and he/she has to select which one is best, or if they have equal quality. Each rater selects from a different randomization of the six methods. The result is a quality score Q for each method, that indicates how often (in %) a method was selected as best, when it was presented to the rater as part of an image pair. No instructions were given to the experts on which features of the image to concentrate on for the quality rating. Inter-rater variability between those two groups was measured using Pearson's r.

4   Results

4.1   B-Spline Fitting Using Data Geometry

Table 1 shows the results when reconstructing US images using the classical B-spline fitting scheme in Eq. (1) with Cartesian and polar grids. MSE, PSNR and SSIM values computed using the original scan converted and interpolated images as reference. Using geometry-adapted (polar) grids, lower MSE and higher PSNR, SSIM and ValL values are obtained suggesting higher quality in the reconstructions compared with Cartesian grids.

Table 1. Mean square error (MSE), Peak Signal to Nose Ratio (PSNR), Structural Similarity Index (SSIM) and Variance of Laplacian (VarL) of B-spline reconstructions with single Cartesian and polar grids.

	MSE	PSNR	SSIM	VarL
Cartesian	395.62 ± 143.30	22.44 ± 1.44	0.76 ± 0.03	113.35 ± 48.05
Polar	$\mathbf{238.99 \pm 162.24}$	$\mathbf{25.01 \pm 2.13}$	$\mathbf{0.78 \pm 0.05}$	$\mathbf{139.24 \pm 51.10}$

4.2   Multi-view Image Compounding

Table 2 reports the VarL values and Q-scores on the six different methods described in Sect. 3. It can be seen, that P2W1 (two view-dependent polar grids

Table 2. Evaluation of multi-view B-spline reconstructions using the Variance of Laplacian (VarL) and a qualitative Q-score obtained by the rating procedure explained in Sect. 3.2. C1: cartesian with one grid; C2: cartesian with two grids; P2: polar with two grids; W0: no weighting; W1: weighting as detailed in Eq. (3).

	C1W0	C1W1	C2W0	C2W1	P2W0	P2W1
VarL	48.6 ± 12.4	93.7 ± 17.4	53.9 ± 14.5	94.9 ± 20.4	92.0 ± 28.1	$\mathbf{139.7 \pm 33.6}$
Q	4.0	26.9	24.6	54.9	71.4	$\mathbf{96.0}$

with data point weighting) received the highest score of Q = 96, i.e. the image obtained by P2W1 was chosen best in 96% of the cases. The "second best" method was P2W0 with Q = 70.7, further demonstrating the importance of the geometry-adapted grids to the final result. This is also reflected in the VarL values. High values, indicating sharper images, are obtained for P2W0 and P2W1.

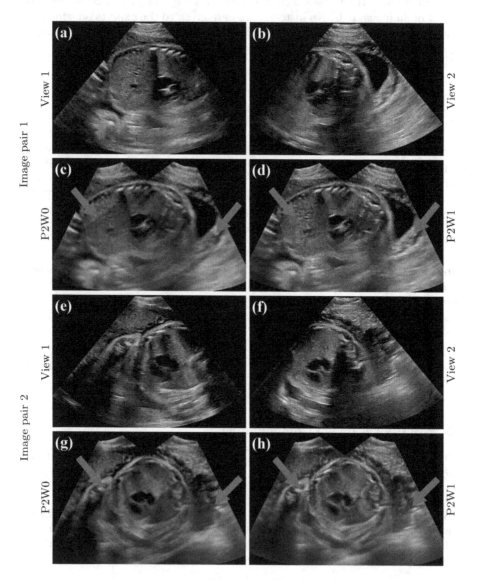

Fig. 3. (a)–(d) Original images of the two views; (e)/(g) compounded image with two polar grids, without data point weighting; (f)/(h) compounded image with two polar grids and data point weighting according to Eq. (3). (Color figure online)

For all grid configurations, the weighting improved both the ValL and Q-scores. While the best ValL values are achieved with all three grid configurations with data point weighting (C1W1: 93.7±17.4, C2W1: 94.0±20.4, P2W1: 139.7± 33.6), the highest Q scores are obtained with the polar grid configuration.

Overall, the inter-rater variability between all raters was low. The correlation measured with Pearson's r is $r = 0.93$ for all experts, when comparing how often each expert selected a specific method as best. The variability when only considering the US engineers was higher ($r = 0.89$) than considering only the clinical experts ($r = 0.95$).

Two examples for the multi-view image compounding are shown in Fig. 3. By combining two views, shadow artifacts are reduced and the field-of-view is extended. By incorporating the data point weighting, artifacts due to varying intensities in both views are reduced (red arrows in Fig. 3 (e)–(h))). Those artifacts were, next to contrast and sharpness of image features, the main aspects the majority of the experts concentrated on for the quality assessment.

5   Discussion and Conclusions

We proposed a method for multi-view US image compounding, that uses multiple geometry-adapted B-spline grids that are simultaneously optimized at multiple levels. Furthermore, we introduced a data point weighting for reducing artifacts arising from different signal intensities in multiple views. Our results on co-planar US image pairs (acquired with two transducers simultaneously and held in the same plane) show that using adapted grids and our proposed weighting system yields better results qualitatively and quantitatively.

Due to the lack of a ground truth for compounded 2D US images, we designed a rating procedure evaluating the quality of the images by experts. There is some disagreement between the VarL scores and the quality rating Q score regarding the different grid and weighting configurations. This raises the question what makes out a good compounding of two US views. The sharpness or blurring, as measured by VarL, is not sufficient to rate the quality of compounding.

Motion was disregarded in our study because by using a rigid physical device, we can ensure that the images are co-planar and the transformation for aligning them is known a priori. However, fetal motion can occur in the small time gap between image acquisition from two transducers. For future work, we plan to incorporate a registration step in our framework to correct for fetal motion.

It is straightforward to generalize our framework to 3D. However, in the real-time 3D mode the frame rate decreases significantly and the assumption of no motion between the two transducer acquisitions does not hold anymore. A registration step becomes inevitable.

The proposed method is not restricted to B-splines for interpolation, and other gridded functions such as Gaussian functions are also possible. The ability to perform multi-view image reconstruction opens several possibilities, for example further reduction of acoustic shadows or other artifacts, or the inclusion of the orientation as additional dimension for image representation [2].

Acknowledgements. This work was supported by the Wellcome Trust IEH Award [102431]. This work was also supported by the Wellcome/EPSRC Centre for Medical Engineering [WT203148/Z/16/Z]. The research was also supported by the National Institute for Health Research (NIHR) Biomedical Research Centre at Guy's and St Thomas' NHS Foundation Trust and King's College London. The views expressed are those of the author(s) and not necessarily those of the NHS, the NIHR or the Department of Health.

References

1. Yao, C., Simpson, J.M., Schaeffter, T., Penney, G.P.: Multi-view 3D echocardiography compounding based on feature consistency. Phys. Med. Biol. **56**(18), 6109–6128 (2011)
2. Hennersperger, C., Baust, M., Mateus, D. Navab, N.: Computational sonography. In: Proceedings of MICCAI, pp. 459–466 (2015)
3. Banerjee, J., et al.: A log-Euclidean and total variation based variational framework for computational sonography. In: Proceedings of SPIE Medical Imaging, vol. 10574 (2018)
4. Lee, S., Wolberg, G., Shin, S.Y.: Scattered data interpolation with multilevel B-splines. IEEE Trans. Vis. Comp. Graph. **3**(3), 228–244 (1997)
5. Ye, X., Noble, J.A., Atkinson, D.: 3-D freehand echocardiography for automatic left ventricle reconstruction and analysis based on multiple acoustic windows. IEEE Trans. Med. Imag. **21**(9), 1051–1058 (2002)
6. Arigovindan, M., Suhling, M., Hunziker, P., Unser, M.: Variational image reconstruction from arbitrarily spaced samples: a fast multiresolution spline solution. IEEE Trans. Imag. Proc. **14**(4), 450–460 (2005)
7. Porras, A.R., et al.: Improved myocardial motion estimation combining tissue Doppler and B-mode echocardiographic images. IEEE Trans. Med. Imag. **33**(11), 2098–2106 (2014)
8. Wang, Z., Bovik, A.C., Sheikh, H.R., Simoncelli, E.P.: Image quality assessment: from error visibility to structural similarity. IEEE Trans. Imag. Proc. **13**(4), 600–612 (2004)
9. Pech-Pacheco, J.L., Cristobal, G., Chamorro-Martinez, J., Fernandez-Valdivia, J.: Diatom autofocusing in brightfield microscopy: a comparative study. Proc. ICPR **3**, 314–317 (2000)

EchoFusion: Tracking and Reconstruction of Objects in 4D Freehand Ultrasound Imaging Without External Trackers

Bishesh Khanal[1,2](✉), Alberto Gomez[1], Nicolas Toussaint[1], Steven McDonagh[2], Veronika Zimmer[1], Emily Skelton[1], Jacqueline Matthew[1], Daniel Grzech[2], Robert Wright[1], Chandni Gupta[1], Benjamin Hou[2], Daniel Rueckert[2], Julia A. Schnabel[1], and Bernhard Kainz[2]

[1] School of Biomedical Engineering and Imaging Sciences,
King's College London, London, UK
bishesh.khanal@kcl.ac.uk
[2] Department of Computing, Imperial College London, London, UK

Abstract. Ultrasound (US) is the most widely used fetal imaging technique. However, US images have limited capture range, and suffer from view dependent artefacts such as acoustic shadows. Compounding of overlapping 3D US acquisitions into a high-resolution volume can extend the field of view and remove image artefacts, which is useful for retrospective analysis including population based studies. However, such volume reconstructions require information about relative transformations between probe positions from which the individual volumes were acquired. In prenatal US scans, the fetus can move independently from the mother, making external trackers such as electromagnetic or optical tracking unable to track the motion between probe position and the moving fetus. We provide a novel methodology for image-based tracking and volume reconstruction by combining recent advances in deep learning and simultaneous localisation and mapping (SLAM). Tracking semantics are established through the use of a Residual 3D U-Net and the output is fed to the SLAM algorithm. As a proof of concept, experiments are conducted on US volumes taken from a whole body fetal phantom, and from the heads of real fetuses. For the fetal head segmentation, we also introduce a novel weak annotation approach to minimise the required manual effort for ground truth annotation. We evaluate our method qualitatively, and quantitatively with respect to tissue discrimination accuracy and tracking robustness.

1 Introduction

Ultrasound (US) is a very widely used medical imaging modality, well known for its portability, low cost, and high temporal resolution. Although the most popular US imaging is 2D B-mode, 3D mode has become an attractive addition providing a larger field of view at an increased frame rate. There is also growing interest in developing low cost 3D US probes [1]. While 2D mode images are

© Springer Nature Switzerland AG 2018
A. Melbourne and R. Licandro et al. (Eds.): DATRA/PIPPI 2018, LNCS 11076, pp. 117–127, 2018.
https://doi.org/10.1007/978-3-030-00807-9_12

usually of higher resolution, 3D mode has the ability to provide better context of the anatomy with smaller number of images. Thus, 3D images could allow easier compounding and field of view extension to capture all the desired anatomy in a single compounded volume.

Volumetric compounding requires the relative transformation between individual volumes. This can be achieved using image registration if the offset is small and assumptions about the spatial arrangement of the volumes hold, e.g., when performing an imaging sweep at constant speed. For large offsets, or random views of a target volume, image registration alone is insufficient and external tracking such as electromagnetic or optical tracking has to be used to establish localisation coherence. External tracking measures absolute transformations between a fiducial marker on the ultrasound probe and a calibrated world coordinate system. Moving targets within a patient cannot be tracked with fiducial markers, computer vision methods that rely on a direct line of sight, or by tracking the probe via external trackers.

An ability to generate high quality compounded volumes of individual fetuses can be useful for retrospective analysis by experts who might not be available, e.g. in rural areas where the live scanning may be performed by non-experts. High quality compounded volumes can also be important in creating US atlases of different fetal organs. For example, it would be desirable to combine all possible views of the brain of single fetus to maximise the information obtained from individual fetal brains. In fetuses of late Gestational ages (GAs), acquiring images from all possible directions requires probe manipulation, incurring large rotation and translational motion. Registration and tracking of images resulting from such constraint-free probe motions is typically highly challenging. A motion-robust and hardware-lean image-based method to compound a large anatomical RoI in real-time is thus highly desired.

Contribution: We propose a novel approach to tackle the tracking problem during 3D fetal US examinations where an application-focused tissue discriminator, based on convolutional neural networks, is integrated into a simultaneous localisation and mapping (SLAM) formulation named EchoFusion. The proposed method yields relative transformations between subsequent volumes, surface reconstruction of the target anatomy, and reconstruction of a compounded volume at the same time. We demonstrate the potential of the proposed approach with experiments for rigid whole body fetal phantom, and for free-hand 4D US covering the head region in real fetuses, without external tracking or a highly restrictive scanning protocol. EchoFusion requires the fetal tissue discriminator to be accurate only in the fetal surface closest to the US probe, allowing the use of: (i) challenging 4D fetal screening US images coming from a very wide range of views, and (ii) weak annotations, enabling large training data at low cost.

Related Work: Extending the FOV by compounding multiple 3D images has been in focus since a wide range of freehand ultrasound probes support 3D images with either matrix array transducers [19] or mechanically steered linear arrays in plane fan mode [5]. Tracking-based methods [3,15] provide good initialisation for a variety of subsequent and task-specific registration methods but often need additional calibration to establish the transformation between object and tracking coordinate system [2]. For rigid non-moving targets, advanced registration strategies can yield good compounding results, given that the acquisition protocol is well defined. For example, [16] uses defined sweeps and multivariate similarity measures in a maximum likelihood framework to mitigate the problem of registration drift observed in earlier, pair-wise registration methods [6]. However, algorithms requiring all the available images simultaneously to estimate transformations cannot be used in real-time applications such as a visual guidance system for non-expert sonographers to receive feedback, during scanning, of the regions already captured.

Recent advances in the robustness of semantic discrimination of tissues in medical images largely enabled by the advent of deep learning, and in SLAM algorithms, provide potential to combine these processes in a reliable fashion. SLAM is known from natural image processing as a powerful tool for indoor [17] and outdoor [8] mapping, location awareness of robots [4] and real-time 3D mesh reconstruction from a stream of RGB images that additionally provide depth information [12]. These techniques have been applied in the medical image analysis community to laparoscopy [19] and movement-based diagnosis [10], but never went beyond RGB (+depth) imaging.

Traditional SLAM methods assume a clear line of sight to map the depth of a scene. However, US images require preprocessing such as segmentation to extract depth of the desired target objects. Convolutional neural networks constitute the state of the art for solving (medical) image segmentation tasks e.g. [9] and have recently shown to be robust for the use in, e.g., fetal screening examinations [20], however only at very young GA when the fetus is fully visible in 3D US volumes. Our work combines fast automatic tissue segmentation that works also on partially visible tissue in later gestation with modern SLAM algorithms. To the best of our knowledge, this is the first time such an approach is proposed.

2   Method

Our approach consists of three main components: **(1)** semantic tissue segmentation, **(2)** transducer to object depth map generation, and **(3)** simultaneous localisation and mapping algorithm. An overview of our approach is shown in Fig. 1.

(1) Semantic tissue discrimination: The objective is to produce a binary segmentation of the target object. For example, for fetal head tracking and reconstruction, the foreground is the fetal head and the remaining structures such as fetal limbs and maternal tissues are background. Fetal segmentation from freehand 4D US can be quite challenging because of the diversity in the image appearance of the same anatomy, cropping due to limited field of view, and the relatively low quality of 4D images compared to 2D images or static 3D volumes. As the images are often corrupted by shadows, fetal body surface at distances far from the transducer cannot be delineated as accurately as surfaces physically nearer to the probe. Thus, in the present work, expert sonographers

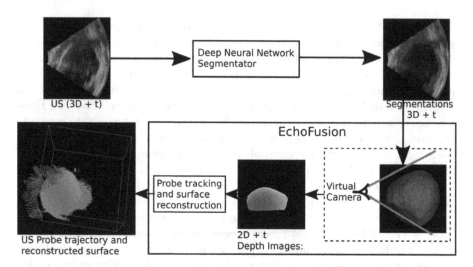

Fig. 1. Overview: Residual 3D U-Net segments each incoming 3D US from which target fetal organ's surface depth is extracted by a virtual camera located at the ultrasound probe. EchoFusion estimates the camera transformation w.r.t previous frame using the incoming depth image and updates the dense surface model.

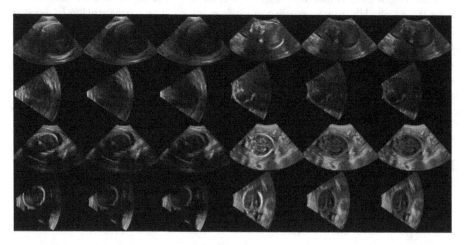

Fig. 2. Four US volumes with input, GT, and predicted volumes (left to right) of two central orthogonal slices. This shows the typical diversity of the input sizes, view direction, partial head views, shadows and US artifacts in the dataset used in our experiments.

delineated the closest surface accurately but approximated the shape of the RoI in the surface further from the probe as shown in Fig. 2.

For semantic segmentation, we use a Residual 3D U-Net architecture which has U-Net structure [13] and is similar to V-net [11] with all convolution layers being replaced by residual-units [7] known to make training more stable. We follow the common strategy whereby skip connections are implemented via concatenation in the up-sampling component of the network and down-sampling is performed with strided convolution (*cf.* max pooling). Each convolutional layer of the original architecture is additionally augmented by a residual block containing two convolutions in a similar fashion to [9]. We employ [16, 32, 64, 128] feature maps per layer and all kernels and feature maps are 3D. Each layer additionally utilizes batch normalization, ReLUs and zero-padding.

For training we draw input training patches of size $64 \times 64 \times 64$ voxels with an equal probability of patches being centered around a voxel from the foreground or background label class. We train to minimize a standard cross-entropy loss using Adam optimization with learning rate of 0.001 and l_2 regularization. Our training imagery is augmented via Gaussian additive noise ($\sigma = 0.02$) with image flipping in each axis.

(2) Transducer distance field generation: Depth images can be generated using a virtual pinhole camera that looks into the 3D segmented model from the same direction as the US probe. All voxels in the output segmentation have known physical co-ordinates with respect to an arbitrary reference point, set as the origin of the world co-ordinate. In the input image volumes, the origin was set to a central point in xz-plane at $y = 0$ making the US probe directed towards positive y-direction and placed $y < 0$. We set a virtual camera that looks towards positive y-axis and along the line $x = z = 0$. The exact position and the view angle of the camera depends on the sector width and sector height of the input 3D US volume. If the camera is too far away, it sees the flat surface at the edge of the US sector. Similarly, if the camera is too close, the FoV is not wide enough and some parts of the tissue region may be missed. In order to estimate an optimal camera position, first we separately compute the intersection and angle between sector lines for the central slices in yz-plane and the central slices in xy-plane as follows:

1. Extract sector mask using thresholding, morphological closing to remove holes.
2. Extract edges using Canny edge detection on the sector mask.
3. Use Hough transform to detect the two sector lines.
4. Compute intersection and angle between the lines found in 3.

Then, the camera distance is set to be the minimum of the two intersection points, and the view angle is chosen to be the wider of the two angles.

(3) Tracking and Reconstruction with EchoFusion: In SLAM [12], a sequence of partial views of a 3D scene captured as 2D RGB images and/or depth images is used to estimate all the relative poses of the camera and reconstruct the 3D scene. Like all SLAM algorithms, we also use only the frontal surface of the 3D scene that are not occluded from the camera view to track and build the 3D scene incrementally. Thus, we use a volumetric surface representation to store global 3D scene as a truncated signed distance function (TSDF) [12] in a predetermined 3D voxel grid. This 3D model is updated with each new incoming depth image by estimating the camera transformation with respect to the previous frame. The algorithm can be outlined as follows:

---

1. From the generated depth image compute the 3D vertex and normals in camera co-ordinate space.

2. The 3D vertex and normals from the previous frame are estimated by ray casting the 3D model built so far from the global camera position estimated from the previous frame.

3. The relative camera transformation is then estimated using Iterative Closest Point (ICP) of the two point sets from the current and the previous frames.

The 3D model gets better and smoother as more consistent data becomes available.

Implementation Details: We adapted an open source implementation[1] of Kinect Fusion [12]. The focal length of the virtual camera can be computed as $f = \frac{w/2}{\tan(\alpha/2)}$, where α is the view angle and w is the image width in pixel co-ordinates. We set depth and RGB image sizes to 480×480. The discriminator model is trained on a Nvidia Titan X GPU with 12 GB of memory. During runtime, the same GPU can be used for inference and EchoFusion, as the inference from the network does not require large resources like in training time. The network was implemented in tensorflow.

3   Experiments and Results

Phantom Data: We use data from a fetal phantom Kyotokagaku UTU-1 at a gestational age of about 20 weeks. The GT segmentation consists of fetal vs. maternal tissue delineation in 28 3D volumes which is randomly split into 24 training samples and 4 validation samples. The GT segmentations include both the fetal head and body as foreground.

Fetal Screening Data: Two expert sonographers delineated 192 US fetal head volumes for training and validation of fetal head segmentation. These 3D images were selected from 4D freehand scanning of 19 different fetuses having GAs in the range of 23–34 weeks with mean (std) age of 30 (2.842) weeks.

The sonographers used MITK [18] to segment six to seven representative slices manually, then performed 3D interpolation from these slices to create a 3D shape. Many of these images contained shadows on the far-field surface, so the manual delineation was done empirically based on the sonographers' anatomical knowledge of the head shape. We split 192 GT data into 184 training and 8 validation images. We then test the trained network only once on a set containing GT segmentations from five fetuses not used in training-validation set.

Evaluation: We use Dice score to evaluate the performance of segmentation quantitatively. Evaluating tracking accuracy is challenging without a ground truth. Surface reconstruction which can be qualitatively observed depends on

---

[1] https://github.com/Nerei/kinfu_remake.

the tracking obtained from the SLAM. To assess the tracking robustness on freehand 4D US stream of the real fetal heads, we test our framework on 37 fetuses and compute the number of tracking losses (i.e. reset of the tracked pose) and the longest sequence without any resets.

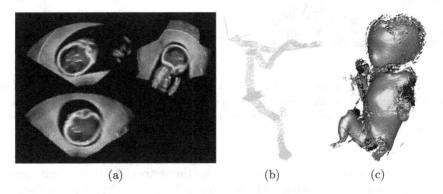

(a)   (b)   (c)

Fig. 3. Orthogonal slices through examples of compounded volumes (a), EchoFusion tracking trajectory (b) and TSDF iso-surface reconstruction (c) for sequences from whole body fetus phantom. The sequence of images of the static phantom were taken with a very wide range of probe directions as seen in the top right slice in (a), and from the trajectory in (b). Limbs are not reconstructed faithfully due to limb information being purposefully discarded at segmentation time.

Results: Table 1 shows quantitative results for segmentation performance on both the phantom and the real fetuses. Since there was only one phantom available which was used to create training and validation set, there is no test set for the phantom. For the real fetuses, test set was created using the same protocol as the training sets but from the fetuses that were not used for training or validation. Although the number of images used for training on the phantom is much smaller than for the real fetuses, the validation set accuracy is higher for the phantom. This is not surprising because the images from the phantom are much less challenging than the real fetuses.

Table 1. Dice scores for real-time semantic tissue discrimination.

Set	images(real)	mean(std)	images(Phantom)	mean(std)
Train	178	0.9408(0.0389)	24	0.9735(0.0125)
Validation	8	0.9217(0.0212)	4	0.9267(0.0074)
Test	26	0.8942(0.0671)	-	-

Figures 3 and 4 show qualitative results after compounding a series of 10–20 EchoFusion-tracked consecutive 3D volume acquisitions from different locations. 3D surface reconstruction in Fig. 3 shows that both the phantom face and body

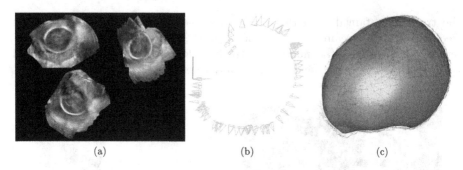

(a)   (b)   (c)

Fig. 4. Orthogonal slices through examples of compounded volumes (a), EchoFusion tracking trajectory (b) and TSDF iso-surface reconstruction (c) for sequences of a real fetal head. Note that the tracking is relative only to the fetal head, and not the other moving maternal and fetal tissues.

which were selected as foreground objects for the segmentation are nicely reconstructed. Similarly, the fetal head in compounded volume in Fig. 4 shows that the sequence of images registered reasonably well although they were taken from a wide range of angles. Table 2 shows EchoFusion tracking performance on 37 fetal sequences of volumes. On average, there were approximately 98 total frames for which the SLAM algorithm lost tracking approximately 5 times. These sequences were obtained by moving the probe in different directions trying to cover the head (skull and face) from all possible directions. The sequences were used as they were acquired without data cleaning, thus containing views which do not show the fetal head and many frames with only partial views of the head region.

Table 2. Robustness with respect to continuously tracked frames for 37 fetuses.

	mean(std)	median	range
Total frames	98.11(54.65)	91	[21, 277]
No. of tracking losses	5.16(3.67)	5	[0, 15]
Longest sequence without tracking loss	40.86(30.85)	31	[4, 152]

4   Discussion

The key contribution of this work is the novel approach to the tracking and compounding problem in freehand 4D US, which constitutes combining the powerful semantic segmentation neural networks with modern SLAM algorithms. Since both of them are very active fields of research, there is a lot of potential to improve EchoFusion for a multitude of applications including compounding, image reconstruction, artefact reduction, super resolution and fetal face biometrics using the resulting dense surface model. Moreover, this method could also allow non-expert to acquire dense data for retrospective evaluation.

The goal of this work was to provide a proof of concept, but clinical translation of this method would require a more extensive quantitative validation of the tracking accuracy, drift over the long sequence, and compare how segmentation accuracy impacts the overall tracking accuracy.

The use of whole body phantom vs fetal head also demonstrates that the top level approach generalises across organs and anatomy as we can train the segmentation network for a desired RoI. However, the current implementation of the SLAM algorithm works only for largely rigid body motion; the static phantom and the fetal head can be reasonably assumed to have mostly rigid body movement with respect to the probe at the semantic level. For non-rigid movements of the fetus such as the whole body or abdomen, the current SLAM component must be replaced with the methods that take dynamic scene changes into account [14]. However, such approaches would still not be robust to sudden movements (*e.g.* kicks) and introduce a significant computational overhead, potentially jeopardizing hard real-time constraints. One approach to tackle this problem is to consider such suddenly moving limbs as background in segmentation so that they are ignored during the tracking and reconstruction. There can still be challenges, (*e.g.* turning the head in the opposite direction and staying there, when reconstructing head/shoulders/torso at once), and is more of an open problem at present. However, being able to focus and compound on quasi-rigid areas like only the head or only abdomen and changing the model depending on target application would already be very valuable e.g., for the creation of fetal brain or abdomen atlases.

5   Conclusion

We have developed a novel approach demonstrating a promising potential for robust segmentation and tracking of fetuses in utero. EchoFusion is versatile and could be applied in any situation where an independently moving target object is occluded by other tissue or material. We have also introduced a way to learn a tissue discriminator from weak annotations in fetal 3D US images and discussed the performance of a Residual 3D U-Net tissue discriminator learning from this data. This discriminator is key to establishing semantics for SLAM-based tracking, which we evaluated on 4D freehand US of a fetal phantom and on real fetuses from screening examinations. In the future, we will perform a more extensive validation of the tracking accuracy, and also find a way to derive robust SDFs from tissue probabilities to exploit the possibilities of dynamic fusion approaches.

Acknowledgements. This work was supported by the Wellcome/EPSRC Centre for Medical Engineering [WT 203148/Z/16/Z], Wellcome Trust IEH Award [102431]. The authors thank Nvidia Corporation for the donation of a Titan Xp GPU.

References

1. Angiolini, F., et al.: 1024-Channel 3D ultrasound digital beamformer in a single 5W FPGA. In: Proceedings of the Conference on Design, Automation & Test in Europe, pp. 1225–1228. European Design and Automation Association (2017)
2. Blackall, J.M., Rueckert, D., Maurer, C.R., Penney, G.P., Hill, D.L.G., Hawkes, D.J.: An image registration approach to automated calibration for freehand 3D ultrasound. In: Delp, S.L., DiGoia, A.M., Jaramaz, B. (eds.) MICCAI 2000. LNCS, vol. 1935, pp. 462–471. Springer, Heidelberg (2000). https://doi.org/10.1007/978-3-540-40899-4_47
3. Octorina Dewi, D.E., Mohd. Fadzil, M., Mohd. Faudzi, A.A., Supriyanto, E., Lai, K.W.: Position tracking systems for ultrasound imaging: a survey. In: Lai, K.W., Octorina Dewi, D.E. (eds.) Medical Imaging Technology. LNB, pp. 57–89. Springer, Singapore (2015). https://doi.org/10.1007/978-981-287-540-2_3
4. Durrant-Whyte, H., Bailey, T.: Simultaneous localization and mapping: part I. IEEE Robot. Autom. Mag. **13**(2), 99–110 (2006)
5. Fenster, A., Downey, D.B.: 3-D ultrasound imaging: a review. IEEE Eng. Med. Biol. Mag. **15**(6), 41–51 (1996)
6. Gee, A.H., et al.: Rapid registration for wide field of view freehand three-dimensional ultrasound. IEEE Trans. Med. Imaging **22**(11), 1344–1357 (2003)
7. He, K., Zhang, X., Ren, S., Sun, J.: Identity mappings in deep residual networks. In: Leibe, B., Matas, J., Sebe, N., Welling, M. (eds.) ECCV 2016. LNCS, vol. 9908, pp. 630–645. Springer, Cham (2016). https://doi.org/10.1007/978-3-319-46493-0_38
8. Heng, L., et al.: Self-calibration and visual SLAM with a multi-camera system on a micro aerial vehicle. Auton. Robot. **39**(3), 259–277 (2015)
9. Kamnitsas, K., et al.: Ensembles of multiple models and architectures for robust brain tumour segmentation. CoRR abs/1711.01468 (2017)
10. Kontschieder, P., et al.: Quantifying progression of multiple sclerosis via classification of depth videos. In: Golland, P., Hata, N., Barillot, C., Hornegger, J., Howe, R. (eds.) MICCAI 2014. LNCS, vol. 8674, pp. 429–437. Springer, Cham (2014). https://doi.org/10.1007/978-3-319-10470-6_54
11. Milletari, F., Navab, N., Ahmadi, S.A.: V-Net: fully convolutional neural networks for volumetric medical image segmentation. In: 2016 Fourth International Conference on 3D Vision (3DV), pp. 565–571. IEEE (2016)
12. Newcombe, R.A., et al.: KinectFusion: real-time dense surface mapping and tracking. In: ISMAR, pp. 127–136. IEEE (2011)
13. Ronneberger, O., Fischer, P., Brox, T.: U-Net: convolutional networks for biomedical image segmentation. In: Navab, N., Hornegger, J., Wells, W.M., Frangi, A.F. (eds.) MICCAI 2015. LNCS, vol. 9351, pp. 234–241. Springer, Cham (2015). https://doi.org/10.1007/978-3-319-24574-4_28
14. Slavcheva, M., Baust, M., Ilic, S.: SobolevFusion: 3D reconstruction of scenes undergoing free non-rigid motion. In: Proceedings of the IEEE Conference on Computer Vision and Pattern Recognition, pp. 2646–2655 (2018)
15. Solberg, O.V., et al.: Freehand 3D ultrasound reconstruction algorithmsa review. Ultrasound Med. Biol. **33**(7), 991–1009 (2007)
16. Wachinger, C., Wein, W., Navab, N.: Three-dimensional ultrasound mosaicing. In: Ayache, N., Ourselin, S., Maeder, A. (eds.) MICCAI 2007. LNCS, vol. 4792, pp. 327–335. Springer, Heidelberg (2007). https://doi.org/10.1007/978-3-540-75759-7_40

17. Whelan, T., et al.: ElasticFusion: dense SLAM without a pose graph. In: Robotics: Science and Systems (2015)
18. Wolf, I., et al.: The Medical Imaging Interaction Toolkit (MITK) a toolkit facilitating the creation of interactive software by extending VTK and ITK
19. Wygant, I.O., et al.: Integration of 2D CMUT arrays with front-end electronics for volumetric ultrasound imaging. IEEE Trans. Ultrason. Ferroelect. Freq. Control **55**(2), 327–342 (2008)
20. Yang, X., et al.: Towards automatic semantic segmentation in volumetric ultrasound. In: Descoteaux, M., Maier-Hein, L., Franz, A., Jannin, P., Collins, D.L., Duchesne, S. (eds.) MICCAI 2017. LNCS, vol. 10433, pp. 711–719. Springer, Cham (2017). https://doi.org/10.1007/978-3-319-66182-7_81

Better Feature Matching for Placental Panorama Construction

Praneeth Sadda[1](✉), John A. Onofrey[1,2], Mert O. Bahtiyar[1,3],
and Xenophon Papademetris[1,2,4]

[1] School of Medicine, Yale University, New Haven, CT 06520, USA
{praneeth.sadda,john.onofrey,mert.bahtiyar,
xenophon.papademetris}@yale.edu
[2] Departments of Radiology and Biomedical Imaging,
Yale University, New Haven, CT 06520, USA
[3] Obstetrics, Gynecology, and Reproductive Sciences,
Yale University, New Haven, CT 06520, USA
[4] Biomedical Engineering, Yale University,
New Haven, CT 06520, USA

Abstract. Twin-to-twin transfusion syndrome is a potentially fatal placental vascular disease of twin pregnancies. The only definitive treatment is surgical cauterization of problematic vascular formations with a fetal endoscope. This surgery is made difficult by the poor visibility conditions of the intrauterine environment and the limited field of view of the endoscope. There have been efforts to address the limited field of view of fetal endoscopes with algorithms that use visual correspondences between successive fetoscopic video frames to stitch those frames together into a composite map of the placental surface. The existing work, however, has been evaluated primarily on *ex vivo* images of placentas, which tend to have more visual features and fewer visual distractors than the *in vivo* images that would be encountered in actual surgical procedures. This work shows that guiding feature matching with deep learned segmentations of placental vessels and grid-based motion statistics can make feature-based registration tractable even in *in vivo* images that have few distinctive visual features.

Keywords: Feature matching · Fetoscopy
Grid-based motion statistics · Mosaic construction
Twin-to-twin transfusion syndrome

1 Introduction

1.1 Twin-to-Twin Transfusion Syndrome

Twin-to-twin transfusion syndrome (TTTS) is a disease of placental vasculature that can affect twin pregnancies. In some twin pregnancies, the two fetuses share a single placenta. It is possible for vascular connections to develop between the

© Springer Nature Switzerland AG 2018
A. Melbourne and R. Licandro et al. (Eds.): DATRA/PIPPI 2018, LNCS 11076, pp. 128–137, 2018.
https://doi.org/10.1007/978-3-030-00807-9_13

portions of the placenta that serve each of the fetuses. When an unequal distribution of blood across these connections leads to a net flow of blood from one twin to the other, the result is TTTS [5]. TTTS can have serious consequences for both twins, including cardiac dysfunction in the twin that serves as a net blood recipient, injury to the central nervous system in the twin that serves as a net donor, and death in either twin [1,5].

While there are several options for managing TTTS, there is only one definitive treatment: fetoscopic laser photocoagulation surgery [4]. In this procedure, a specialized endoscope known as a fetoscope is inserted through an incision in the maternal abdominal wall and then into the uterus. Once in the uterus, the fetoscope is used to inspect blood vessels on the surface of the placenta. Any problematic vascular connections that are found are cauterized with a laser. This procedure is illustrated in Fig. 1.

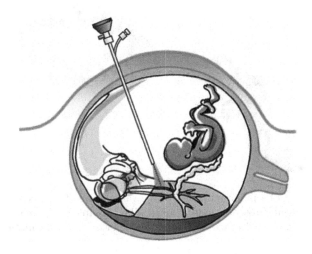

Fig. 1. A diagram of fetoscopic laser photocoagulation surgery for twin-to-twin transfusion syndrome by Luks [8]. Pictured are twin fetuses, each within their own amniotic sac. There is a single, shared placenta with problematic vascular connections that allow a net flow of blood from the donor fetus (left) to the recipient fetus (right). An endoscope (top) is used to inspect the placental vasculature and find problematic connections. When such connections are found, they are cauterized with a laser (center).

The challenges of fetoscopic laser photocoagulation are well described in the literature [12–14]. The problematic placental vascular formations cannot be visualized preoperatively with ultrasound or magnetic resonance imaging. They must therefore be identified intraoperatively using a fetoscope. This is made difficult, however, by the turbidity of amniotic fluid. The turbid nature of amniotic fluid not only reduces the clarity of the fetoscopic image, but also makes it impossible for the fetoscope's attached light source to reliably illuminate structures that are more than a few centimeters away. The fetoscope must therefore be kept close to the placental surface, but this has the effect of reducing the field of view.

The distance across the placental vascular network (i.e. the distance from one twin's umbilical cord to the other) can be several dozen times the diameter of the fetoscope's field of view. As the surgeon can only see a small fraction of the placental surface at any given time, he or she must create a mental map of the relevant placental anatomy in real time and must rely on landmarks from this mental map in order to remain oriented as the surgery progresses. The high cognitive burden that fetoscopic laser photocoagulation surgery places on the surgeon increases the risk of error, which in the worst case can lead to the failure to identify and cauterize one or more vascular malformations, thereby necessitating a follow-up surgery. There has been interest in reducing the cognitive burden on the surgeon by replacing the surgeon's mental map-making process with computer software that performs a similar task.

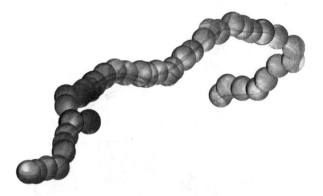

Fig. 2. An example of a panoramic view of the vasculature of a placenta that was created by concatenating fetoscopic video frames. This example was manually constructed from 30 min of fetoscopic footage from a fetoscopic laser photocoagulation surgery.

1.2   Prior Work

In the existing literature on placental panorama construction, by far the most common approach is to extract visual frame-to-frame correspondences and use those correspondences to calculate a homography from one frame to the other [3,7,10,14]. Such approaches consist of a four step process: *(i)* using a feature detector to select key points from within an image; *(ii)* converting the high-dimensional raw pixel data of the image regions surrounding each key point into lower-dimensional vectors with the use of a feature description algorithm; *(iii)* matching the key points from one image with key points from the other, usually via a nearest-neighbor criterion on the key points' associated feature descriptors; and *(iv)* calculating a homography from the coordinates of the matched key points. The two most popular feature matching and description algorithms in the existing literature on placental panorama construction are the Scale-Invariant Feature Transform (SIFT) and its derivation, Speeded Up Robust Features (SURF).

To the best of the authors' knowledge, all placental panorama construction studies to date have been evaluated primarily on *ex vivo* images [3,10,12–14] or images of placental phantoms [7]. *Ex vivo* images of placentas, however, tend to have more visual features and fewer visual distractors than *in vivo* images [6,7]. Blood vessels are identifiable in both *ex vivo* and *in vivo* images, but *ex vivo* feature-rich backgrounds whereas *in vivo* images tend to have backgrounds that are almost entirely featureless (Fig. 3).

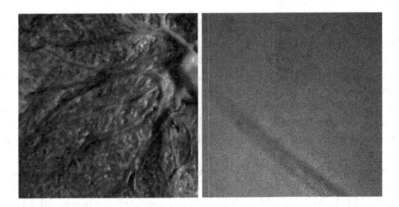

Fig. 3. Blood vessels are visible in both *ex vivo* and *in vivo* images of placentas. *Ex vivo* images, however, are rich in background features while *in vivo* images often have backgrounds that are entirely devoid of features. In the *in vivo* image, the guide light for the cautery laser is visible in the upper center area. The guide light moves along with the fetoscope, so it is not suitable as a landmark for registration.

Gaisser *et al.* [7] simulated *ex vivo* and *in vivo* settings using a placental phantom and found that the performance of SIFT and SURF feature detectors could fall dramatically in the translation to *in vivo*. When applied to images from an *in vivo* setting with amniotic fluid of a yellow coloration, SIFT detected 73% fewer features than it did in an *ex vivo* setting. SURF detected 45% fewer features. The results reported by Gaisser *et al.* suggest that the underlying issue in registering *in vivo* placental images is a dearth of high-quality key points. If few key points are repeatable between different *in vivo* views of the same portion of a placenta, then there will be few matches. A homography calculated from a small number of matches will be highly sensitive to false or outlier matches. Furthermore, if the number of matches is low enough it will not be possible to compute a homography at all. Bian *et al.* [2] argue, however, that in many feature matching tasks, the underlying issue is not that there is a lack of good key points or good matches, but that standard matching techniques have difficulty distinguishing good matches from bad matches. It follows that better algorithms for determining matches between feature descriptors may be able to produce more accurate homographies for registering *in vivo* placental images into a panoramic map. In this work, we show that by extending the matching algorithm beyond the typical nearest-neighbor approach, it is possible to extract meaningful matches between *in vivo* placental images even with low-quality key points and to exceed the accuracy of registrations produced with SURF and SIFT feature matching.

2   Methods

2.1   Feature Matching

Bian *et al.* [2] argue that when feature matching fails to produce sufficient matches, the underlying issue is often not a lack of good matches, but difficulty in distinguishing good matches from bad matches. In other words, when scoring matches (which is typically done by calculating the distance between the feature descriptors of the two matched key points), there tends to be a significant overlap between the score distribution of true matches and the score distribution of false matches. Setting a high minimum threshold for the match score minimizes the number of false positive matches but also eliminates many true matches.

Feature descriptor distance is not the only method for scoring matches. Bian *et al.* [2] propose scoring feature matches using the observation that true matches are likely to be neighbored by other true matches whereas false matches are more frequently found in isolation. Preliminary feature matches are first generated using the traditional nearest-neighbor approach. One image in the pair is then divided into a regularly spaced grid. A secondary score for a match that falls within the i-th cell of the first image and the j-th cell of the second is calculated as follows:

$$S_{i,j} = |X_{i,j}| - 1$$

where $X_{i,j} = \{x_1, x_2, x_3, ..., x_n\}$ is the union of matches found in the i-th cell of the first image and the j-th cell of the second. This secondary score is used to determine which cells in the first image are paired with which cells in the second. A constraint is then enforced in which key points within a given cell in the first image must match to its paired cell in the second image. Bian *et al.* refer to this approach as grid-based motion statistics (GMS). We apply a GMS match refinement step after the initial nearest-neighbor matching.

2.2   Feature Detection and Description

When matching key points with GMS, the quantity of key points is more important than their quality. We therefore use a feature detector that can generate a large number of key points: the AGAST corner detector [9]. We further increase the number of key points by lowering the AGAST detection threshold to zero and disabling the suppression of non-max corners. Although GMS is predicated on the notion that low quality key points can produce useful matches, it remains a fact that not all key points are of equal value. *In vivo* fetoscopic images are filled with visual distractors such as the glare effects and floating debris in the amniotic fluid. These visual distractors are not useful for computing homographies between placental images.

In Sadda et al. [11], we showed that a neural network could be trained to segment blood vessels in *in vivo* placental images with human-level accuracy. We repurpose the segmentations produced by this trained neural network as a key point filter. Only key points that fall on a placental blood vessel are used; all other key points are discarded. The remaining key points are described with SIFT descriptors and matched with a nearest-neighbors approach. The matches are then refined with GMS.

2.3 Image Acquisition

In vivo placental images were acquired to evaluate the registration approach described in this paper. Intraoperative videos of ten fetoscopic laser coagulation surgeries performed at Yale-New Haven Hospital were obtained in a process approved by an institutional review board. All ten videos were recorded using a Karl Storz miniature 11540AA endoscope with incorporated fiber optic light transmission. 544,975 video frames were collected in total, accounting for approximately five hours of video. These video frames were cropped and downscaled from an initial resolution of 1920×1080 pixels to a resolution of 256×256 pixels.

3 Results and Discussion

3.1 Synthetic Registration Task

188 video frames were extracted from the dataset of *in vivo* fetoscopic videos described in Sect. 2.3. Each image was randomly rotated between 0 and 360 degrees, translated by up to 64 pixels (one-quarter of the side-length of the viewport) along each axis, and perspective-warped by displacing each of the four corners of the image by up to 20 pixels.

Table 1. The results of the synthetic registration task described in Sect. 3.1. Fetoscopic video frames were distorted with randomly generated homographies. Various feature matching algorithms were used to recover the homographies. Each algorithm was evaluated in terms of success rate, defined as the percentage of image pairs for which the algorithm found enough matches to compute a homography, and transformation error, defined as the mean distance between a grid of points transformed by the ground truth homography and the same points transformed by the recovered homography.

Algorithm	Transformation error (pixels)	Success rate
SIFT	143.3 ± 366.2	49.5%
SURF	60.3 ± 65.7	85.1%
AGAST + SIFT + GMS	3.2 ± 5.5	100.0%

Various feature matching algorithms were used to recover the homography between the original image and the distorted image. Each algorithm was evaluated in terms of success rate, defined as the percentage of image pairs for which

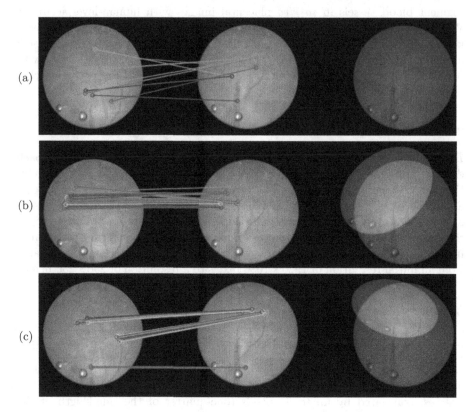

Fig. 4. An example from the natural registration task described in Sect. 3.2. The lower part of image A (left column) contains the upper ends of the blood vessels found in image B (center column). A composite image (right column) is created by overlaying the registered image A on top of image B. Several algorithms were compared: (a) Standard SURF key point detection and feature description yields a high ratio of false matches to total matches. This leads to image A being misregistered to such an extent that it falls completely outside of the composite image. (b) AGAST key point detection, SURF feature description, and GMS refinement of matches yields fewer false matches, but many of these matches are centered in a largely featureless background region. This leads to a number image A being registered to approximately the correct region of B but without proper alignment of the blood vessels in A to the corresponding vessels in B. (c) By using a deep-learned vessel segmentation algorithm, it is possible to limit AGAST key points to those that fall on blood vessels. This results in the algorithm correctly registering image A to the upper portion of image B. There are enough true matches for RANSAC-based homography estimation to identify and eliminate the false matches at the bottom of the images. The blood vessels in A are correctly aligned to the corresponding vessels in B.

the algorithm found enough matches to compute a homography, and transformation error, defined as the mean distance between a grid of points transformed by the ground truth homography and the same points transformed by the recovered homography. The results are summarized in Table 1.

The registration task in this experiment is admittedly trivial: since one image in each pair is a direct geometric transformation of the other image, a feature descriptor that lacked any invariance to lighting, illumination, or noise would in theory be able to generate matches across the images. However, this task is sufficient to show that the standard usage patterns of SIFT and SURF are unsuitable even for very trivial registration problems involving *in vivo* placental images. These methods fail to produce enough matches to compute a homography in a significant fraction of cases, and even when they can produce homographies, the homographies are of much lower quality than those produced by matching AGAST features with GMS.

3.2   Natural Registration Task

22 image pairs were selected from the dataset of *in vivo* fetoscopic videos described in Sect. 2.3. Each pair consisted of two images that depicted overlapping segments of the same vascular formation. To ensure that the frames were sufficiently different to make registration a nontrivial task, pairs were selected such that the video frames in each pair were acquired a minimum of 20 seconds apart. One image from each pair was manually rotated, translated, and perspective warped in an image editing program until it was aligned with the other image. The transformation

Table 2. The results of the natural registration task described in Sect. 3.2. Each algorithm was evaluated in terms of success rate, defined as the percentage of image pairs for which the algorithm found enough matches to compute a homography, and transformation error, defined as the mean distance between a grid of points transformed by the ground truth homography and the same points transformed by the recovered homography. The algorithms are as follows: *(i)* SIFT key point detection and SIFT feature description; *(ii)* SURF detection and description; *(iii)* SURF with key points filtered by a deep learned mask; *(iv)* SURF with a deep learned mask and with the Hessian threshold for detection reduced to zero; *(v)* AGAST feature detection, SIFT feature description and subsequent refinement of matches with grid-based motion statistics (GMS); and *(vi)* the AGAST/SIFT/GMS pipeline with the addition of a deep mask.

Algorithm	Transf error (pixels)	Success rate
SIFT	97.1 ± 34.6	72.72%
SURF	158.9 ± 143.9	100.00%
SURF + Deep Filter	223.5 ± 215.7	40.90%
SURF (0 threshold) + Deep Filter	118.9 ± 57.0	100.00%
AGAST + SIFT + GMS	45.6 ± 21.2	100.00%
AGAST + Deep Filter + SIFT + GMS	55.1 ± 32.1	100.00%

matrix corresponding to the concatenation of these editing operations was saved as the ground truth homography for that image pair.

Several feature matching and algorithms were executed on each image pair in an effort to recover the ground truth homography from visual correspondences. Each algorithm was evaluated in terms of success rate and transformation error, as defined in Sect. 3.1. The results are summarized in Table 2 and Fig. 4. Standard SIFT and SURF approaches perform poorly. SIFT fails to produce enough key point matches to produce a homography in over one quarter of cases. SURF is able to generate a homography more frequently, but the homographies that it produces have a high transformation error relative to the ground truth. One might expect that applying the deep learned vessel segmentations as a key point mask would help eliminate matches to visual distractors and increase match quality. However, applying deep filtering to SURF further reduces the number of available features, and lowering the Hessian threshold to increase the number of SURF features does not lead to better matches. Matching with GMS consistently produces the best registrations.

Adding a deep filter to GMS matching slightly increases the average transformation error. This is the result of images in which there is a single, linear blood vessel. As the deep filter limits key points to those that lie on a blood vessel, it causes the set of matched points in such images to be almost co-linear, and even slight deviations in the positions of matched key points can have a large effect on the computed homography if they are orthogonal to the axis of the lone blood vessel.

4   Conclusion

Prior research into the construction of panoramic maps of the placenta has made great strides in processing *ex vivo* placental images. Given that the ultimate goal is to use this technology intraoperatively, the next step is to extend existing techniques to handle the more complicated domain of *in vivo* images. However, the most common technique for panorama construction in the existing literature, nearest neighbor matching of SIFT and SURF features, gives unsatisfactory results even for very trivial registration tasks involving *in vivo* images. Feature matching with *in vivo* placental images is difficult because placental images lack a rich variety of visually distinct features. The appearance of one blood vessel on a placenta is not necessarily significantly different from the appearance of another blood vessel a centimeter away, and this leads to a high rate of false matches. In this work, we demonstrate that the paucity of visually distinct features is not necessarily a limiting factor in the registration of *in vivo* images. By using matching algorithms that impose a structure on matched elements – in this case a grid-based locality constraint – it is possible to significantly improve the quality of feature matches and the resulting image registrations.

Acknowledgements. This work was supported by the National Institutes of Health grant number T35DK104689 (NIDDK Medical Student Research Fellowship). The authors would like to thank Andreas Lauritzen for his assistance with data collection.

References

1. Bahtiyar, M.O.: The North American fetal therapy network consensus statement: prenatal surveillance of uncomplicated monochorionic gestations. Obstet. Gynecol. **125**(1), 118–123 (2015)
2. Bian, J., Lin, W.Y., Matsushita, Y., Yeung, S.K., Nguyen, T.D., Cheng, M.M.: GMS: grid-based motion statistics for fast, ultra-robust feature correspondence. In: 2017 IEEE Conference on Computer Vision and Pattern Recognition (CVPR), pp. 2828–2837, July 2017
3. Daga, P., et al.: Real-time Mosaicing of Fetoscopic Videos Using SIFT, vol. 9786, pp. 9786–9786-7 (2016)
4. Emery, S.P., Bahtiyar, M.O., Moise, K.J.: The North American fetal therapy network consensus statement: management of complicated monochorionic gestations. Obstet. Gynecol. **126**(3), 575–584 (2015)
5. Faye-Petersen, O.M., Crombleholme, T.M.: Twin-to-twin transfusion syndrome. NeoReviews **9**(9), e380–e392 (2008)
6. Gaisser, F., Peeters, S.H.P., Lenseigne, B., Jonker, P.P., Oepkes, D.: Fetoscopic panorama reconstruction: moving from ex-vivo to in-vivo. In: Valdés Hernández, M., González-Castro, V. (eds.) Medical Image Understanding and Analysis, pp. 581–593 (2017)
7. Gaisser, F., Peeters, S.H.P., Lenseigne, B.A.J., Jonker, P.P., Oepkes, D.: Stable image registration for in-vivo fetoscopic panorama reconstruction. J. Imaging **4**(1), 24 (2018)
8. Luks, F.: Schematic Illustration of Endoscopic Fetal Surgery for Twin-to-Twin Transfusion Syndrome, December 2009
9. Mair, E., Hager, G.D., Burschka, D., Suppa, M., Hirzinger, G.: Adaptive and generic corner detection based on the accelerated segment test. In: Daniilidis, K., Maragos, P., Paragios, N. (eds.) ECCV 2010. LNCS, vol. 6312, pp. 183–196. Springer, Heidelberg (2010). https://doi.org/10.1007/978-3-642-15552-9_14
10. Peter, L., et al.: Retrieval and registration of long-range overlapping frames for scalable mosaicking of in vivo fetoscopy. Int. J. Comput. Assist. Radiol. Surg. **13**(5), 713–720 (2018)
11. Sadda, P., Onofrey, J., Imamoglu, M., Papademetris, X., Qarni, B., Bahtiyar, M.O.: Real-time computerized video enhancement for minimally invasive fetoscopic surgery. Laparoscopic Endoscopic Robot. Surg. **1**, 27–32 (2018)
12. Tella-Amo, M., et al.: A combined EM and visual tracking probabilistic model for robust mosaicking: application to fetoscopy. In: The IEEE Conference on Computer Vision and Pattern Recognition (CVPR) Workshops, June 2016
13. Tella-Amo, M., et al.: Probabilistic visual and electromagnetic data fusion for robust drift-free sequential mosaicking: application to fetoscopy. J. Med. Imaging **5**(2), 5–16 (2018)
14. Yang, L., et al.: Towards scene adaptive image correspondence for placental vasculature mosaic in computer assisted fetoscopic procedures. Int. J. Med. Robot. Comput. Assist. Surg. **12**(3), 375–386 (2016)

Combining Deep Learning and Multi-atlas Label Fusion for Automated Placenta Segmentation from 3DUS

Baris U. Oguz[1], Jiancong Wang[1], Natalie Yushkevich[1], Alison Pouch[1], James Gee[1], Paul A. Yushkevich[1], Nadav Schwartz[2], and Ipek Oguz[1(✉)]

[1] Penn Image Computing and Science Laboratory (PICSL),
Department of Radiology, University of Pennsylvania,
Philadelphia, PA, USA
ipek@cs.unc.edu
[2] Maternal and Child Health Research Program, Department of OBGYN,
University of Pennsylvania, Philadelphia, PA, USA

Abstract. In recent years there is growing interest in studying the placenta in vivo. However, 3D ultrasound images (3DUS) are typically very noisy, and the placenta shape and position are highly variable. As such, placental segmentation efforts to date have focused on interactive methods that require considerable user input, or automated methods with relatively low performance and various limitations. We propose a novel algorithm using a combination of deep learning and multi-atlas joint label fusion (JLF) methods for automated segmentation of the placenta in 3DUS images. We extract 2D cross-sections of the ultrasound cone beam with a variety of orientations from the 3DUS images and train a convolutional neural network (CNN) on these slices. We use the prediction by the CNN to initialize the multi-atlas JLF algorithm. The posteriors obtained by the CNN and JLF models are combined to enhance the overall segmentation performance. The method is evaluated on a dataset of 47 patients in the first trimester. We perform 4-fold cross-validation and achieve a mean Dice coefficient of 86.3 ± 5.3 for the test folds. This is a substantial increase in accuracy compared to existing automated methods and is comparable to the performance of semi-automated methods currently considered the bronze standard in placenta segmentation.

1 Introduction

Adverse pregnancy outcomes such as preeclampsia and intrauterine growth restriction contribute to perinatal morbidity and mortality. Given mounting evidence [1–3] that placental abnormalities are related to such outcomes, placental morphometry has recently become major foci of study. Ultrasound imaging is the most common modality to study the placenta in clinical settings due to its low cost, wide availability and ease of acquisition. 2D and 3D ultrasound have

© Springer Nature Switzerland AG 2018
A. Melbourne and R. Licandro et al. (Eds.): DATRA/PIPPI 2018, LNCS 11076, pp. 138–148, 2018.
https://doi.org/10.1007/978-3-030-00807-9_14

been used to study early, in utero placental size and morphology in relation to birthweight and preeclampsia [14,16]. While placental biometry may be helpful in clinical care [15], there is currently no clinical tool to evaluate placental morphology due to the lack of automated segmentation methods.

Automated quantification of the placenta from 3D ultrasound images (3DUS) is challenging. 3DUS images are prone to high levels of speckle noise, and the contrast between the placenta and uterine tissue is especially weak in early pregnancy. Additionally, the position of the placenta with respect to the amniotic sac is highly variable which makes it difficult to even detect the placenta automatically, much less determine its precise boundaries. In particular, placentas can be positioned anteriorly or posteriorly to the amniotic sac. Maternal habitus and fetal shadowing artifacts can further obscure the placenta boundary, especially in posterior placentas. The size and shape of the placenta are variable, and uterine contractions can dramatically affect the shape of the placenta.

Many current techniques for placental segmentation from 3DUS rely on user input to overcome these challenges. These include the commercial VOCAL software (GE Healthcare) and a random-walker (RW) algorithm [4,17]. Such interactive methods are time-consuming, subjective and prone to intra- and interobserver variability, which makes automated methods more attractive. Only 4 fully automated approaches have been proposed to date.

1. A recurrent neural network [19]. While this is a more general-purpose segmentation framework that aims to segment not just the placenta but also the gestational sac and the fetus, the placenta segmentation accuracy achieved with this method is rather limited (average Dice of 0.64 is reported in [19]).
2. A multi-atlas label fusion algorithm [10]. Since this is a registration-based method, it suffers from registration initialization robustness issues. The fully automated version of the algorithm relies on initialization based on the ultrasound cone beam, but is limited to anterior placentas (mean Dice of 0.83 in anteriors reported in [10]). For generalization to non-anterior placentas, manual initialization on a 2D slice is required to guide the registration [11].
3. A deep convolutional neural network (CNN), DeepMedic [8]. The "ground truth" segmentations are produced via the RW algorithm [17], as opposed to fully manual expert annotations used in other studies. While this algorithm is readily applicable to anterior and posterior placentas, the performance leaves room for improvement (median Dice of 0.73 reported in [8]).
4. An improved version of [8], with a 3D fully convolutional network (OxNNet) [9]. Perhaps the most distinguishing aspect of this paper is the significantly larger amount of training data. They utilize 2400 labelled 3DUS images in a 2-fold cross validation setup. They report a mean Dice score of 0.81. Like [8], this used the results of the random walker algorithm as "truth".

We propose a novel technique that combines the strengths of the deep learning and multi-atlas label fusion (MALF) approaches for fully automated segmentation of the placenta from 3DUS images. MALF methods require good registration initialization and have limited performance in hard-to-register patches such as thin features and low-contrast boundaries. CNN's [6] are more robust to such problems but tend to be noisier, and are hard to train in 3D given the sparsity of training data in medical image analysis; as such, their results can lack 3D shape context. Triplanar CNN's were studied in [12] as a workaround. In our proposed algorithm, we begin with a 2D CNN to construct an initial prediction and we leverage the rotational ambiguity of the ultrasound cone beam for an innovative data augmentation strategy. Next, we deploy a MALF algorithm using the CNN results to initialize the registrations. We use a second-tier model to combine the posterior maps from the CNN model and the MALF method.

2   Methods

Our algorithm begins with pre-processing and extracting 2D slices from the 3DUS images and trains a convolutional neural network (CNN) with online random augmentation to create an initial prediction in 3D. Next, multi-atlas joint label fusion (JLF) is applied on the CNN output to construct an alternative prediction. The predictions from CNN and JLF are combined via a second tier random forest (RF) model to obtain the final segmentation result (Fig. 1a).

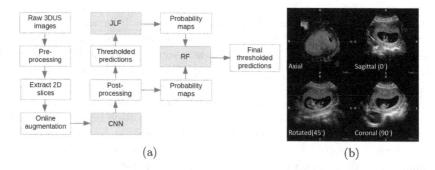

(a)   (b)

Fig. 1. (a) Workflow of our algorithm. (b) Placenta cross-sections from various views.

2.1   Dataset, Pre-processing and Augmentation

Our dataset consists of first trimester 3D US images from 47 subjects with singleton pregnancies, acquired with GE Voluson E8 ultrasound machines. 28 subjects had anterior placentas, and 19 had posterior placentas. Each image has isotropic resolution (mean: 0.47 mm, min: 0.35 mm, max: 0.57 mm). Each image was manually segmented by N.Y.. under the supervision of N.S., who has over 10 years of experience in prenatal ultrasound imaging and who has segmented 100's of placentas for other research endeavors. The ITK-SNAP software[1] was used for segmentation. The main metric for evaluating the pipeline is the Dice overlap between automated results and these manual segmentations.

---

[1] www.itksnap.org.

26 of the 47 subjects were imaged twice within the same session. Patients were allowed to move around between the two acquisitions. These secondary images were used in a reproducibility experiment, described in Sect. 2.6 below.

The images in our dataset have various dimensions and may contain sizable blank spaces around the edges. Thus, the images are cropped to a 3D bounding box of the ultrasound cone beam (automatically, by simply thresholding at 0), and downsampled to standard dimensions (128^3).

We extract 2D slices from the original 3D images and train a CNN with 2D convolutions. Our experiments showed that the axial view presents little information to the CNN regarding the placenta. Therefore, we extract slices only in the sagittal ($0°$) and coronal ($90°$) planes, and a $45°$ plane between them. This leads to a stack of $128 \times 3 = 384$ slices per subject, along 3 different orientations. Given the rotational ambiguity of the ultrasound probe, these 3 orientations contain similar cross-sections of the placenta (Fig. 1b).

To further mitigate the impact of a small training dataset, we use online random augmentation. Various transforms are applied to each 2D slice before it is seen by the CNN. These transforms consist of horizontal/vertical flipping, 2D translation, 2D rotations (in-plane), and scaling. Whether each transformation is applied, and if relevant its magnitude, is determined randomly. Translation magnitudes are between $-5/+5$ pixels (image size is 128×128). In-plane rotation amount is between $-15/+15°$. Scaling is performed by zooming in 0–10%.

2.2 Convolutional Neural Network

Typical CNN's for classification tasks [6] contain 3 main types of layers: (1) Convolutional layers extract local features by sliding a kernel (aka filter) over the input image to compute a feature map. (2) Pooling layers downsample the feature maps obtained by the convolutional layer, commonly applying a function like max, mean, sum, etc. (3) Fully connected layers consolidate the features from convolutional and pooling layers, and output probabilities for each class.

The strength of convolutional layers and CNN's comes from their ability to preserve spatial relationships in the input images. The main parameters that affect the performance of a convolutional layer are the kernel size, the strides, and the number of feature maps. Kernel size and strides are often chosen empirically in relation to the input image dimensions. The number of feature maps determines the number of trainable parameters in the layer and must be chosen with consideration of under/over-fitting.

Initial convolutional layers usually extract low-level features such as edges, corners, etc. Successive layers build on top of previously extracted feature maps and discover higher-level features significant for the task. Pooling layers condense the information from convolutional layers, by retaining whether a feature is present in the active kernel window, but dismissing the exact location within the kernel. While this quality is favorable in many vision tasks where the goal is to detect a higher level entity (cat, car, face) in the image, in our preliminary experiments we found that using pooling layers degrades the mean Dice results of CNN predictions. This might be because the task of segmentation requires a decision for each voxel in the input. However, further investigation remains for future work; in the work presented here, pooling layers were not used.

U-net [13] proposes a multi-channel approach to the problem of retaining location information. They use max-pooling layers for downsampling but still present the unpooled feature maps to the final convolution by side channels. In our approach, we utilize convolutional layers with larger strides instead of pooling, to retain the benefit of condensing feature information, while keeping the location information intact. This effectively downsamples the feature maps from the convolutional layers, while preventing systematic loss of information.

Fully connected layers are used when the dimensions of the output are much smaller relative to the input (classification, bounding box locations, etc.). In the segmentation task, the dimensions of the output are identical to that of the input. To reach the required output dimensions from the downsampled feature maps, we apply upsampling via transposed convolution (aka deconvolution) layers.

Our CNN architecture consists of 23 layers in total: 1 batch normalization, 15 ordinary convolutions (1×1 strides), 3 downsampling convolutions (2×2 strides), 3 upsampling deconvolutions (2×2 strides), and 1 sigmoid output (Fig. 2). All the kernels we use in the convolutional layers have the dimensions of 3×3, and ReLU was used as activation function in all intermediate layers.

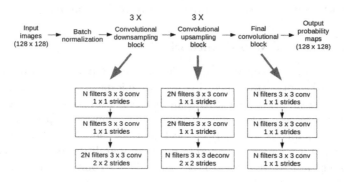

Fig. 2. Our CNN architecture contains 23 layers in total: 1 normalization + 18 convolutional + 3 deconvolutional + 1 sigmoid. There are 2,730,627 trainable parameters.

In the training phase, we use 384 2D slices for each subject (128 each from $0°$, $45°$, and $90°$ orientations), and train a single CNN. In the prediction phase, we produce 4 probability maps for each 2D slice, by flipping the slice horizontally and vertically. The mean of the 4 orientations is used as the prediction for that slice. For each subject, we predict for the three orientations above, obtaining three 3D probability maps. To provide an initialization for the JLF step, we take the mean of these three maps and binarize by a threshold.

The CNN code is implemented on the Python/Numpy stack. We used TensorFlow for the CNN backend and Keras as a higher level frontend. The CNN training is run on a machine with 4x Nvidia GTX-1080Ti GPUs. The online random augmentation is performed on the CPU, in parallel to the CNN working on the GPU. One epoch of training takes around 2–3 min, the final model at 35 epochs lasts around 90 min. Due to our cross-validation setup, we trained 4 such models, one for each fold. The total time for the CNN part of the pipeline takes around 8 h including pre/post processing. The prediction phase is much faster and completes within minutes for the entire dataset.

2.3   Joint Label Fusion (JLF)

Registration-based segmentation methods are popular in medical image analysis. In the simplest form, an atlas image is created via manual annotation. This atlas image is registered deformably to the target image, and the segmentation of the target is calculated by applying the same deformation to the atlas annotation. This single atlas method does not generalize well, due to the large variability in shape, size, and location of anatomical structures. The next evolution of this method utilizes multiple atlases instead of a single one [5]. Each atlas produces a solution to the target image, and these solutions are combined in a label fusion step. The fusion is typically based on a weighted voting scheme, usually taking into consideration the similarity of each atlas to the target image.

Specifically, we use the publicly available JLF approach [18] for label fusion, which jointly estimates the weights for all available atlases, minimizing the redundancy from correlated atlases. These weights are given by $w_x = \frac{M_x^{-1} 1_n}{1_n^t M_x^{-1} 1_n}$, where $1_n = [1; 1; \ldots; 1]$ is a vector of size n and t stands for transpose. The dependency matrix M is estimated by $M_x(i,j) = [|A^i(N(x)) - T(N(x))| \cdot |A^j(N(x)) - T(N(x))|]^\beta$, where $|A^i(N(x)) - T(N(x))|$ is the vector of absolute intensity difference between a warped atlas A^i and the target image over a local patch $N(x)$ centered at x and $\cdot$ is the dot product. β is a model parameter. Default values were used for all parameters in the JLF implementation [18].

All registrations were done using the open source greedy package[2]. We use the binary prediction from the CNN as a mask to guide the affine registrations, which use the SSD metric. The subsequent deformable registrations do not use a mask as the affine registration provides a stable enough initialization; the normalized cross correlation (NCC) metric is used with a $4 \times 4 \times 4$ patch size.

2.4   Combining CNN and JLF Results

Our CNN step produces 3 probability maps for each subject (for $0°$, $45°$, and $90°$ orientations). We average and threshold these to provide input for the JLF step. We obtain another probability map from the JLF, ending up with 4 maps. Simply averaging these maps offers limited Dice improvement over the individual probability maps. To extract more information from the 4 maps, we utilize a second tier model. This model takes the 4 probabilities for each pixel and additional statistical features (min, mean, max, stdev, max-min) to produce a final probability. We use a random forest model with 50 trees and max depth of 6.

---

[2] https://sites.google.com/view/greedyreg/home.

2.5   Experimental Methods for Cross-Validation

Given the relatively small dataset, we opted for a two-tiered 4-fold cross-validation (cv) scheme. At each cv step of the 1st tier, we used 3 folds for training a CNN, and the last fold for testing, ending up with 4 CNN's. Each of these CNN's use identical architecture and parameters, to prevent overfitting to a single test fold.

These unseen test fold predictions are then used as a registration mask in the JLF part of the pipeline. For each subject, the manual segmentations from all training subjects are used as atlases (i.e., training), using the same train/test split as the CNN folds. Thus, for each of the test folds, we end up with 3 probabilities (for $0°$, $45°$, and $90°$ orientations) from a CNN and the JLF probability.

To train the 2nd tier RF, we apply an inner 4-fold cv to each test fold from the CNN/JLF tier, for a total of 16 RF models with identical parameters. Finally, we approximate the performance on an independent validation set by taking the mean of the results from the 16 unseen test folds of the 2nd tier inner cv.

2.6   Reproducibility Experiment

During the recording of 3DUS images, movements of the subject and the fetus, specific position of the ultrasound probe, and other factors may result in significant variations in image appearance. 26 of the 47 subjects in our dataset have secondary images taken within the same session, which we use to test the reproducibility of our algorithm. In this experiment, we trained our CNN model on the 21 subjects with only one image. We performed the JLF step with using only these 21 subjects as atlases. We trained the RF models via an inner 4-fold on these 21 subjects. Using this pipeline trained on the disjoint set of 21 subjects, we segmented the placenta for the 26 test subjects, 2 segmentations for each subject (one per image). We calculated the volume of the segmentations, and evaluated the correlation of volume between the pairs of images.

3   Results

Our results are summarized in Fig. 3. The proposed combination of CNN and JLF results via a second tier RF model outperforms the individual methods.

		CNN	JLF	CNN+JLF+RF	p-value (CNN, CNN+JLF+RF)	p-value (JLF, CNN+JLF+RF)
ANTERIOR	Mean ± SD	0.849 ± 0.064	0.849 ± 0.058	0.875 ± 0.052	6.37E-05	5.82E-08
	[Min, Max]	[0.693, 0.925]	[0.700, 0.927]	[0.764, 0.943]		
POSTERIOR	Mean ± SD	0.821 ± 0.048	0.812 ± 0.059	0.846 ± 0.052	1.73E-03	9.69E-05
	[Min, Max]	[0.749, 0.907]	[0.677, 0.898]	[0.730, 0.924]		
OVERALL	Mean ± SD	0.838 ± 0.060	0.834 ± 0.060	0.863 ± 0.053	2.47E-07	7.64E-11
	[Min, Max]	[0.693, 0.925]	[0.677, 0.927]	[0.730, 0.943]		

Fig. 3. Dice scores for test folds. P-values from paired two-tailed t-tests are reported.

These differences were found to be highly significant ($p < 0.001$) in paired two-tailed t-tests. We note that all compared methods have lower performance in the posterior placentas where fetal shadowing artifacts are common. Qualitative results are shown in Fig. 4. The reproducibility results are shown in Fig. 5-a.

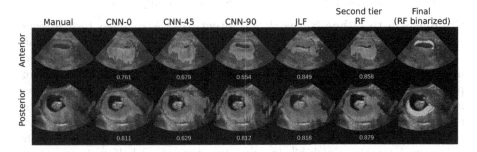

Fig. 4. Qualitative results from an anterior and a posterior subject. In the first subject, CNN models are erroneously drawn to bright regions, but the JLF accurately captures the placenta. In the second subject, JLF oversegments the placenta due to weak boundaries, but CNN models capture the correct result. In both subjects, the second-tier RF model effectively combines the two approaches.

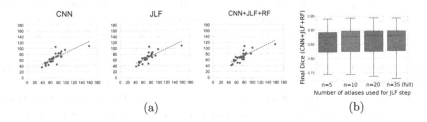

Fig. 5. (a) Test-retest volumes (measured in ml) at each stage of our pipeline are shown for 26 pairs of images. The Pearson correlation coefficient between volume test-retest measurements was 0.786 for CNN, 0.787 for CNN+JLF, and 0.797 for the final (CNN+JLF+RF) method. Final correlation was 0.848 when one outlier was removed, and 0.874 when 3 outliers were removed. (b) Final Dice scores with various number of atlases for the JLF step. The differences between using the entire training fold ($n = 35$) and only 5 randomly selected subjects were minimal (0.859 vs. 0.863).

4   Discussion

Our Findings. Our combined approach utilizes both the automated power of CNN's and the 3D context of multi-atlas label fusion. Both methods have their strengths and weaknesses, and our second tier RF model effectively blends their results into a more accurate and robust final prediction. Our results (0.863 mean

Dice overall) provide a substantial improvement over existing automated methods (mean Dice of 0.81 reported in [9], median Dice of 0.73 reported in [8], mean Dice of 0.64 reported in [19], mean Dice of 0.83 reported for anterior-only placentas in [10]), and are comparable to the performance of semi-automated methods (mean Dice scores of 0.80 reported in [11] and 0.86 reported in [17]), which require manual input and may have reproducibility issues.

Comparison to Other Network Architectures. A common task in computer vision is classification, including binary, multi-class and multi-label problems. In these settings, the output is one or more ordinal labels for each input image. Common architectures for this task contain convolution and downsampling layers in the first half of the network. The second half contains fully connected dense layers, producing predicted labels from the inner representation of the first half. Image segmentation differs from classification, requiring an output for each input voxel. Thus, most common architectures are variations of the fully convolutional network [7]. In this setup, the second half contains upsampling layers, producing a full size prediction from the inner representation. Our CNN is also based on this architecture. In the downsampling layers, we used strided convolutions, which produced better results in our experiments than the pooling approach. We also experimented with U-net [13] style side channels, but that also did not provide much improvement, and extended training time. A formal comparison of these alternative architectures remains as future work.

2D vs. 3D CNNs. In recent years, CNN's have consistently shown high performance in many visual learning tasks, especially thriving on large amounts of training data. The medical imaging field, in contrast, typically has much less data available. Our annotated 3DUS dataset consists of 47 subjects, which is significantly low in quantity when compared to general image datasets containing multi-million labelled images used for more general CNN tasks. It is difficult to obtain large amounts of labeled placenta images, since the segmentation needs to be manually created by expert annotators in a time-consuming process.

While it is possible to train a CNN on 3D images using 3D convolutions, our dataset size is too small to fully take advantage of such an approach. Training 3D CNN's also requires much larger computational resources compared to 2D CNN's. Therefore, we opted for using 2D CNNs on slices from the 3DUS images. Evidently, this leads to a loss of 3D context. We mitigated this shortcoming by extracting 2D slices from three different axises. We also applied random online augmentation during training to further increase the variance in the dataset.

Number of Atlases Needed for MALF. MALF is computationally intensive. The runtime grows linearly with each atlas and each test subject, since each pair needs to be registered. In our dataset consisting of 47 subjects, using all train-fold subjects ($n = 35$) as atlases took around 1000 CPU-hours on a computer cluster, utilizing up to 25 CPUs in parallel. This is longer than the CNN training time. More importantly, in a real-life application, the CNN only needs to be trained once whereas the atlas registrations are needed for each new test subject. This causes a bottleneck for the practical applicability of our method.

We hypothesized that the main benefit from the JLF step in this application is the access to 3D context, which can be gained from just a handful of atlases. This is unlike other applications where a large set of atlases are needed to adequately represent the underlying distribution of image appearance. To test this hypothesis, we experimented with using a small random subset of subjects in the train fold as atlases, instead of all of them. The results for utilizing 5-10-20 atlases are given in Fig. 5-b. While using the full train fold as atlases gives the best results, the mean Dice when using only 5 randomly chosen subjects is still very closely comparable (0.8588 vs. 0.8631). This finding supports our hypothesis. It also reinforces the main idea behind our approach, which is combining two methodologically different approaches to produce a more robust segmentation. Running the JLF step with even just 5 atlases provides considerable improvement in the Dice scores while reducing the runtime substantially.

Acknowledgments. This work was funded by the NICHD Human Placenta Project (U01 HD087180) and NIH grants R01 EB017255, R01 NS094456 and F32 HL119010.

References

1. Baptiste-Roberts, K., Salafia, C.M., Nicholson, W.K., Duggan, A., Wang, N.Y., Brancati, F.L.: Gross placental measures and childhood growth. J. Matern.-Fetal Neonatal Med. **22**(1), 13–23 (2009)
2. Barker, D.J., Bull, A.R., Osmond, C., Simmonds, S.J.: Fetal and placental size and risk of hypertension in adult life. BMJ **301**(6746), 259–262 (1990)
3. Biswas, S., Ghosh, S.K.: Gross morphological changes of placentas associated with intrauterine growth restriction of fetuses: a case control study. Early Hum. Dev. **84**(6), 357–362 (2008)
4. Collins, S.L., Stevenson, G.N., Noble, J.A., Impey, L.: Rapid calculation of standardized placental volume at 11 to 13 weeks and the prediction of small for gestational age babies. Ultrasound Med. Biol. **39**(2), 253–260 (2013)
5. Iglesias, J.E., Sabuncu, M.R.: Multi-atlas segmentation of biomedical images: a survey. Med. Image Anal. **24**(1), 205–219 (2015)
6. Krizhevsky, A., Sutskever, I., Hinton, G.E.: ImageNet classification with deep convolutional neural networks. In: NIPS, pp. 1097–1105 (2012)
7. Long, J., Shelhamer, E., Darrell, T.: Fully convolutional networks for semantic segmentation. In: IEEE CVPR, pp. 3431–3440 (2015)
8. Looney, P., et al.: Automatic 3D ultrasound segmentation of the first trimester placenta using deep learning. In: IEEE ISBI, pp. 279–282 (2017)
9. Looney, P., et al.: Fully automated, real-time 3D ultrasound segmentation to estimate first trimester placental volume using deep learning. JCI Insight (2018)
10. Oguz, I., et al.: Fully automated placenta segmentation from 3D ultrasound images. In: Perinatal, Preterm and Paediatric Image Analysis, PIPPI Workshop, MICCAI (2016)
11. Oguz, I., et al.: Semi-automated 3DUS placental volume measurements with minimal user interaction. The American Institute of Ultrasound in Medicine (2018)

148 B. U. Oguz et al.

12. Prasoon, A., Petersen, K., Igel, C., Lauze, F., Dam, E., Nielsen, M.: Deep feature learning for knee cartilage segmentation using a triplanar convolutional neural network. In: Mori, K., Sakuma, I., Sato, Y., Barillot, C., Navab, N. (eds.) MICCAI 2013. LNCS, vol. 8150, pp. 246–253. Springer, Heidelberg (2013). https://doi.org/10.1007/978-3-642-40763-5_31

13. Ronneberger, O., Fischer, P., Brox, T.: U-Net: convolutional networks for biomedical image segmentation. In: Navab, N., Hornegger, J., Wells, W.M., Frangi, A.F. (eds.) MICCAI 2015. LNCS, vol. 9351, pp. 234–241. Springer, Cham (2015). https://doi.org/10.1007/978-3-319-24574-4_28

14. Schwartz, N., Quant, H.S., Sammel, M.D., Parry, S.: Macrosomia has its roots in early placental development. Placenta **35**(9), 684–690 (2014)

15. Schwartz, N., Wang, E., Parry, S.: Two-dimensional sonographic placental measurements in the prediction of small-for-gestational-age infants. Ultrasound Obstet. Gynecol. **40**(6), 674–679 (2012)

16. Schwartz, N., et al.: Placental volume measurements early in pregnancy predict adverse perinatal outcomes. Am. J. Obstet. Gynecol. **201**(6), S142–S143 (2009)

17. Stevenson, G.N., Collins, S.L., Ding, J., Impey, L., Noble, J.A.: 3-D ultrasound segmentation of the placenta using the random walker algorithm: reliability and agreement. Ultrasound Med. Biol. **41**(12), 3182–3193 (2015)

18. Wang, H., Yushkevich, P.: Multi-atlas segmentation with joint label fusion and corrective learning–an open source implementation. Front. in Neuroinf. **7**, 27 (2013)

19. Yang, X., et al.: Towards automatic semantic segmentation in volumetric ultrasound. In: Descoteaux, M., Maier-Hein, L., Franz, A., Jannin, P., Collins, D.L., Duchesne, S. (eds.) MICCAI 2017. LNCS, vol. 10433, pp. 711–719. Springer, Cham (2017). https://doi.org/10.1007/978-3-319-66182-7_81

LSTM Spatial Co-transformer Networks for Registration of 3D Fetal US and MR Brain Images

Robert Wright[1(✉)], Bishesh Khanal[1], Alberto Gomez[1], Emily Skelton[1], Jacqueline Matthew[1], Jo V. Hajnal[1], Daniel Rueckert[2], and Julia A. Schnabel[1]

[1] School of Biomedical Engineering and Imaging Sciences,
King's College London, London, UK
`robert.wright@kcl.ac.uk`
[2] Department of Computing, Imperial College London, London, UK

Abstract. In this work, we propose a deep learning-based method for iterative registration of fetal brain images acquired by ultrasound and magnetic resonance, inspired by "Spatial Transformer Networks". Images are co-aligned to a dual modality spatio-temporal atlas, where computational image analysis may be performed in the future. Our results show better alignment accuracy compared to "Self-Similarity Context descriptors", a state-of-the-art method developed for multi-modal image registration. Furthermore, our method is robust and able to register highly misaligned images, with any initial orientation, where similarity-based methods typically fail.

1 Introduction

Registration, the process of aligning images, is an important technique which allows visual inspection and computational analysis of images in a common coordinate system. For fetal abnormality screening, registered Magnetic Resonance (MR)/Ultrasound (US) images may assist diagnosis as the two modalities capture complementary anatomical information. For example, in the fetal brain, MR images have better contrast between important structures such as cortical Grey Matter (GM) and White Matter (WM), whereas the higher spatial resolutions of US gives better discrimination between fine structures such as the septum pellucidum and the choroid plexus [7].

A voxel-wise image similarity measure or cost function is commonly used in medical imaging to register images. This function quantifies the alignment of images, where an extremum gives the optimum alignment between images. Unfortunately, image similarity-based methods are ill-suited to the challenging task of US/MR image registration as there is no global intensity relationship between the two modalities. Primarily this is due to the imaging artefacts present in US images, such as view-dependent shadows, speckle noise, anisotropy, attenuation, reverberation and refraction. Popular similarity measures developed specifically for other multi-modal registration problems in the past, such

© Springer Nature Switzerland AG 2018
A. Melbourne and R. Licandro et al. (Eds.): DATRA/PIPPI 2018, LNCS 11076, pp. 149–159, 2018.
https://doi.org/10.1007/978-3-030-00807-9_15

as Normalised Mutual Information (NMI), often fail, even with a good initialisation [12].

Consequently, an alternative approach has arisen for registration of images with non-global intensity relationships whereby image intensities are first transformed to a modality independent representation. These are typically derived from hand-crafted descriptors which capture structural information from images such as edges and corners. Representations used by previous authors include local gradient orientation [4], local phase [9] and local entropy [16]. Notably, [5] use the concept of self-similarity, computing the similarity of small image patches in a local neighboured within an image, which achieved state-of-the-art performance on a challenging US/MRI registration dataset. Another approach to this problem is modality synthesis, which aims to transform image intensities from one modality to another allowing the registration task to be treated as a mono-modal problem. [7] made use of this approach to register the fetal brain imaged by US and MR for the first time.

More recently, deep neural networks have been applied to the problem of registration. Two common strategies for registration with deep learning include estimating a similarity measure [2,15] and predicting transformations directly [1,13]. An advantage of the first approach is that it allows established transformation models and optimizers to be used, however, this could be a hindrance if the learnt similarity function is not smooth or convex. The second approach, predicting the parameters of a transformation model directly, is receiving more research focus recently as it allows more robust transformation estimates.

1.1 Proposed Method

In this work, we adopt a deep learning approach to tackle the challenging task of paired 3D MR/US fetal brain registration. Our Long Short-Term Memory (LSTM) network simultaneously predicts a joint isotropic rescaling plus independent rigid transformations for both MR/US images, aligning them to a dual-modality spatio-temporal atlas (Sect. 2.6). Transformation estimates are refined iteratively over time, allowing for higher accuracy. For this, we extend the iterative spatial transformer [8] for co-transformation of multiple images (see Fig. 1). The main contributions of this work are as follows:

- A network architecture inspired by spatial transformer networks [6] for group-wise registration of images to a common pose.
- A loss function which encourages convergence and fine alignment of images.

2   Methods

2.1   Overview

The spatial transformer module [6] allows geometric transformation of network inputs or feature maps within a network, conditioned on the input or feature

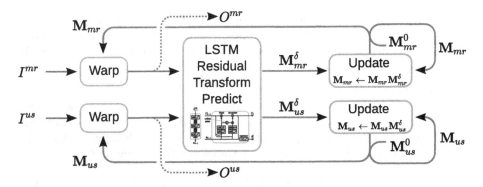

Fig. 1. Proposed LSTM spatial co-transformer for coalignment of 3D MR/US images. Flow of image intensities is shown in blue while flow of transformation parameters is shown in red. An LSTM network predicts residual transformations $\mathbf{M}_{mr}^{\delta}$, $\mathbf{M}_{us}^{\delta}$ conditioned on the current warped images O^{us}, O^{mr}, iteratively refining their alignment. (Color figure online)

map itself. Importantly, the spatial transformer module is differentiable, allowing end-to-end training of any network it is inserted into. This allows reorientation of an image into a canonical pose, simplifying the task of subsequent layers. [8] proposed an elegant iterative version of the spatial transformer that passes composed transformation parameters through the network instead of warped images, preserving image intensities until the final transformation. The same geometric predictor with a much simpler network architecture can be used in a recurrent manner, for more accurate alignment.

In this work, we propose a novel extension the "recurrent/LSTM spatial co-transformer", which allows simultaneous transformation of multiple images to a common pose. Commonly, registration algorithms estimate a warp from one image (the source) towards another (the target). However, we found that fine alignment is more easily learnt between images in a common pose. Thus, we simultaneously co-align pairs of MR/US images to a common atlas-space (Sect. 2.6), which will also facilitate future computational image analysis.

Additionally, we propose an LSTM-based parameter prediction network (Fig. 2) and a temporally varying loss function (Sect. 2.5) for more accurate alignments.

2.2 Recurrent Spatial Co-transformer

The recurrent spatial co-transformer consists of three main components: (1) the warper, (2) the residual parameter prediction network and (3) the composer. The first component, the warper, is the computational machinery needed to transform an image and does not contain any learnable parameters. For simplicity of discourse, we treat this as a single function f_{warp} and refer the reader to [6] for a detailed description of grid transformation and differentiable interpolation. The second component, the parameter prediction network, $f_{predict}$, predicts residual transformations conditioned on the current warped output images. Finally, the third component, the composer, updates the transformation estimates. The recurrent spatial co-transformer iterates between three steps, which will now be described in more detail.

Step 1 - Image Warping. For iteration t, Let $\mathcal{I} = (I^0, I^1, \dots, I^N)$ denote an N-tuple of input images, $\Theta_t = (\theta_t^0, \theta_t^1, \dots, \theta_t^N)$ denote an N-tuple of corresponding transformation estimates and $\mathcal{O}_t = (O_t^0, O_t^1, \dots, O_t^N)$ denote an N-tuple of corresponding warped output images. Then each input image I^i is first warped independently given its last transformation estimate θ_{t-1}^i

$$O_{t-1}^i = f_{warp}(I^i, \mathbf{G}, \theta_{t-1}^i) \quad \forall i \in [1, \dots, N]. \tag{1}$$

Here, $\mathbf{G} = [\mathbf{g}_1, \dots, \mathbf{g}_g] \in \mathbb{R}^{4 \times g}$ is a matrix of homogeneous grid coordinates.

Step 2 - Residual Parameter Prediction. Warped images $\mathcal{O}_{t-1}$ are concatenated along the channel axis and passed as a single tensor to $f_{predict}$ which simultaneously predicts an N-tuple of corresponding residual transformations $\Delta_t = (\delta_t^0, \delta_t^1, \dots, \delta_t^N)$

$$\Delta_t = f_{predict}(O_{t-1}^0 \frown O_{t-1}^1 \frown \dots \frown O_{t-1}^N). \tag{2}$$

$f_{predict}$ can take any form but typically consists of a feed-forward network with several interleaved convolutional and max pooling layers followed by a fully connected layer and a final fully connected regression layer with the number of units equalling the number of model parameters.

Step 3 - Parameter Composition. Finally, each transformation estimate θ_{t-1}^i, is composed with its residual transformation estimate δ_t^i, yielding a new transformation estimate θ_t^i

$$\theta_t^i = f_{update}(\theta_{t-1}^i, \delta_t^i) \quad \forall i \in [1, \dots, N]. \tag{3}$$

The composition function f_{update} will vary depending on the transformation model. For example, if θ parametrises a homogeneous transformation matrix, f_{update} would be matrix multiplication.

2.3   LSTM Spatial Co-transformer

For more accurate parameter prediction, we propose an LSTM network architecture for $f_{predict}$. LSTMs are an extremely powerful network architecture capable of storing information in a cell state allowing them to learn long term dependencies in sequential data much better than recurrent neural networks. For this we modify the prediction function $f_{predict}$ (Eq. 2) so that it now takes a feature vector $\mathbf{x}_t$, and a cell state vector $\mathbf{c}_t$

$$\Delta_t = f_{predict}(\mathbf{x}_t, \mathbf{c}_t), \text{ where } \mathbf{x}_t = f_{extract}(O_{t-1}^0 \frown O_{t-1}^1 \frown \dots \frown O_{t-1}^N). \tag{4}$$

Here $f_{extract}$ is a function that extracts the feature vector $\mathbf{x}_t$ from the concatenation of the output images, $O_{t-1}^0 \frown O_{t-1}^1 \frown \dots \frown O_{t-1}^N$. For this, we chose a neural network with a series of convolutions and max pooling operations followed by a flattening procedure (see Fig. 2 for a schematic, however any network architecture may be used that produces a vector). At each iteration t, the cell state $\mathbf{c}_t$ is updated by a linear blend of the previous cell state $\mathbf{c}_{t-1}$ and a vector of candidate values $\tilde{\mathbf{c}}_t$ [3]

$$\mathbf{c}_t = \mathbf{f}_t \odot \mathbf{c}_{t-1} + (1 - \mathbf{f}_t) \odot \tilde{\mathbf{c}}_t. \tag{5}$$

Here, $\odot$ is the Hadamard or element-wise product and $\mathbf{f}_t$ is the forget mask, a real valued vector that determines which information is forgotten from the cell state and which candidate values are added. We define $\mathbf{f}_t$ as the result of a single function f_{forget} that takes the extracted feature vector $\mathbf{x}_t$ and also the previous cell state $\mathbf{c}_{t-1}$. We implement both the forget and candidate functions as a sequence of two dense layers with weight matrices $\mathbf{W}_{f1}$, $\mathbf{W}_{f2}$ and $\mathbf{W}_{c1}$, $\mathbf{W}_{c2}$, respectively

$$\mathbf{f}_t = f_{forget}(\mathbf{c}_{t-1}, \mathbf{x}_t) = \sigma(\mathbf{W}_{f2}.\max(\mathbf{W}_{f1} \cdot [\mathbf{c}_{t-1}, \mathbf{x}_t], 0)), \tag{6}$$

$$\tilde{\mathbf{c}}_t = f_{candidate}(\mathbf{c}_{t-1}, \mathbf{x}_t) = \tanh(\mathbf{W}_{c2}.\max(\mathbf{W}_{c1} \cdot [\mathbf{c}_{t-1}, \mathbf{x}_t], 0)). \tag{7}$$

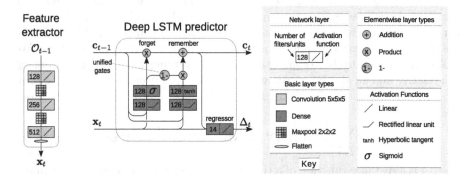

Fig. 2. LSTM parameter prediction architecture for rigid alignment of MR/US images. The image feature extractor encodes a dual-channel image as a vector that is passed into an LSTM network which predicts a residual transformation. Fourteen parameters are predicted: three for rotation, three for translation and one for isotropic scale, per modality (note, weights for scaling are shared between modalities).

2.4   Rigid Parameter Prediction

For rigid coalignment, our network predicts seven residual update parameters per image: an isotropic log scaling s, three rotation parameters r_x, r_y, r_z and three translation parameters t_x, t_y, t_z. Here, $[r_x, r_y, r_z]$ gives an axis of rotation, while $\phi = \|[r_x, r_y, r_z]\|_2$, gives the angle of rotation. Note, weights are shared between images for scaling parameters. Our transformation parameters now become rigid transformation matrices $\delta_t = \mathbf{M}_t^\delta$, $\theta_t = \mathbf{M}_t$. Note, for simplicity, transformations $\mathbf{M}$ are applied to the target grid $\mathbf{G}$ before resampling, i.e. the inverse transformation. For consistency, we define $\mathbf{M}^\delta$ as the inverse update and $(\mathbf{M}^\delta)^{-1}$ as the forward update. Learning a series of forward update transformations is inherently easier for the network, thus we post-multiply the current transformation matrix by the residual matrix, $\mathbf{M} \leftarrow \mathbf{M}\mathbf{M}^\delta$. This is equivalent to updating the forward transformation as follows $\mathbf{M}^{-1} \leftarrow (\mathbf{M}^\delta)^{-1}\mathbf{M}^{-1}$. The forward update transformation is composed as a translation, followed by a rotation, followed by an isotropic rescaling, $(\mathbf{M}^\delta)^{-1} = \mathbf{SRT}$. In practice, we predict the inverse of the update directly by reversing the composition and inverting the operations $\mathbf{M}^\delta = \mathbf{T}^{-1}\mathbf{R}^{-1}\mathbf{S}^{-1}$.

2.5   Training and Loss Function

Let $\mathbf{X} = \{\mathcal{I}_0, \mathcal{I}_1, \dots, \mathcal{I}_n\}$ denote a training set of n aligned image tuples. Images in the training set are initially aligned to a common pose (in our case we affinely align our MR and US images to a dual-modality atlas, see Sect. 2.6). For each training iteration, an image tuple is selected $\mathcal{I} = (I^0, I^1, \dots, I^N)$ and each image I^i is transformed by a randomly generated matrix $\mathbf{D}^i$, before being fed into the network. $\mathbf{D}^i$ incorporates an affine augmentation (shared across the input tuple) and an initial rigid disorientation. For augmentation, we randomly sample and compose a shearing, an anisotropic scaling and an isotropic scaling. For disorientation, we compose a random rotation and translation. Crucially, the use of a recurrent network allows us to back-propagate errors through time. We took advantage of this by designing a temporally varying loss function comprising of a relative and an absolute term, which allows our network to learn a long term strategy for alignment. For k alignment iterations of N images, we define our loss

$$\mathcal{L} = \sum_{i=1}^{N} \sum_{t=1}^{k} d(\mathbf{M}_t^i \, \mathbf{D}^i) / d(\mathbf{M}_{t-1}^i \, \mathbf{D}^i) + \lambda \frac{t}{k} \, d(\mathbf{M}_t^i \, \mathbf{D}^i). \tag{8}$$

Here, d is a distance function of a transformation matrix from the identity and λ is a weighting between the loss terms. The first loss term rescales distance errors $d(\mathbf{M}_t^i \, \mathbf{D}^i)$, relative to the previous distance error, $d(\mathbf{M}_{t-1}^i \, \mathbf{D}^i)$. This encourages the network to learn fine alignments and convergence. Note, $d(\mathbf{M}_{t-1}^i \, \mathbf{D}^i)$ is treated as a constant here. The second term penalises the absolute error with increasing weight, encouraging initial exploration but still penalising poor final alignments. The distance function $d(\mathbf{M})$ is computed by first decomposing matrix $\mathbf{M}$ into a isotropic scale s, a translation vector $\mathbf{t}$ and a rotation matrix $\mathbf{R}$. We then compute $d(\mathbf{M})$ as a sum of separate distance measures for each of these components

$$d(\mathbf{M}) = d_{scale}(s) + d_{rotate}(\mathbf{R}) + d_{translate}(\mathbf{t}), \quad \text{where} \quad d_{translate}(\mathbf{t}) = \|\mathbf{t}\|_2 \,,$$

$$d_{scale}(s) = \mu \, |\log(s)| \quad \text{and} \quad d_{rotate}(\mathbf{R}) = \frac{1}{g} \sum_{i=1}^{g} \|\mathbf{g}_i - \mathbf{R}\mathbf{g}_i\|_2 \,. \tag{9}$$

Here, μ weights d_{scale} relative to the other two distance measures. Rotation distance, d_{rotate}, is given by the mean distance between transformed grid points $\mathbf{Rg}_i$ and their initial locations $\mathbf{g}_i$. This gives a natural weighting between translation and rotation components.

2.6 Joint Affine MR/US Spatio-Temporal Atlas (Ground Truth)

We followed the approach of [14], by constructing average image intensity templates for each week of gestation (20–31 weeks), from 166 3D reconstructed MR/3D US image pairs. A set of templates was constructed for each modality separately with a final registration step between templates to establish correspondences across modalities. This process comprised of three parts: (1) manual reorientation (2) age-dependant template bootstrapping and (3) unified template bootstrapping. All images were carefully manually reoriented to a standard pose with the yz plane aligned with the brain midline and the top of the brain stem centred at the origin. Averaging reoriented image intensities yielded an initial template estimate which was refined using a bootstrapping procedure. This involved alternating between two steps: (1) affinely registering images to the current template and (2) averaging registered image intensities. The bootstrapping procedure was then repeated between templates to establish correspondences across time. MR templates were constructed first, allowing us to fix the shearing and scaling parameters for US template construction. For US registration, we restrict the optimisation to three degrees of freedom, rotation around x, and translation along y and z, thus respecting the manual definition of the midline. With additional masking, this allowed robust registration of US images for template construction using [10].

3   Results and Discussion

3.1   Alignment Error

To demonstrate the accuracy of our method (LSTM ST) we compute registration errors with respect to two ground truth alignments: the first, derived from our spatio-temporal atlas and the second, derived from anatomical landmarks picked by clinical experts (fourteen per image), which offers an unbiased alternative. For comparison, two image similarity-based registration methods were chosen, NMI with block-matching (NMI+MI) [10] and self-similarity context descriptors with discrete optimisation (SSC+DO) [5]. Both of these methods were developed for robust registration and have been used for multi-modality registration tasks previously. To compare the accuracy of the methods and also their ability to register highly misaligned images, we created three test sets with different ranges of disorientation: [3–5°, 3–5 mm], [30–60°, 10–20 mm] and [90–180°, 30–50 mm].

As we can see from Table 1 our method outperforms both similarity-based methods for all disorientation levels and both ground truth datasets. Furthermore, our method converges to the same alignment for each image pair, irrespective of initial orientation and positioning, which explains the very similar mean errors seen for the three disorientation levels. Conversely, similarity-based methods failed to register images for higher levels of disorientation. All pairs of images registered by our method were visually inspected and a reasonable alignment was found in all cases (see Fig. 3 for example alignments). The worst

Table 1. Mean alignment error. Mean rotation and translation errors over our test set are shown for three automated registration methods, relative to two ground truth alignments.

(a) Atlas-based ground truth alignment						
Disorientation		NMI+BM		SSC+DO		LSTM ST
3–5°	3–5mm	23.00°	3.49 mm	4.08°	1.01 mm	2.97°	0.63 mm
30–60°	10–20 mm	42.11°	5.26 mm	36.62°	3.97 mm	2.94°	0.63 mm
90–180°	30–50 mm	131.25°	9.18 mm	129.74°	13.01 mm	2.91°	0.62 mm
(b) Landmark-based ground truth alignment						
Disorientation		NMI+BM		SSC+DO		LSTM ST
3–5°	3–5 mm	23.84°	3.57 mm	5.49°	1.73 mm	4.06°	1.60 mm
30–60°	10–20 mm	42.58°	5.22 mm	35.16°	4.11 mm	4.03°	1.60 mm
90–180°	30–50 mm	131.70°	8.98 mm	131.28°	11.68 mm	4.03°	1.60 mm

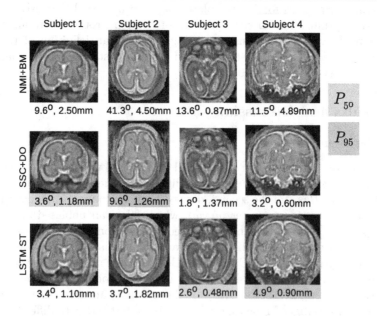

Fig. 3. Median (blue) and 95th percentile (red) alignments by rotation error for SSC+DO and LSTM ST. Alignments for other methods are shown for comparison. Each column shows the same MR image for a subject from our test set with its corresponding US image thresholded, colour-mapped, overlayed and aligned, by each of the automated methods. (Color figure online)

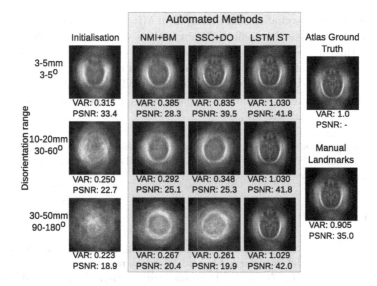

Fig. 4. Template sharpness. Templates are constructed by averaging image intensities for US images registered to an MR template via their corresponding MR images (see Sect. 3.2). Higher Variance of the Laplacian (VAR) indicates sharper templates and better registration accuracy, while higher Peak Signal-to-Noise Ratio (PSNR) indicates greater similarity with the atlas ground truth template.

rotation and translation errors seen were $7.9°$ and 1.8 mm respectively, showing our method is relatively robust.

3.2 Mean Templates

We construct US mean templates by first registering each US image to its corresponding MR image, rigidly, then affinely transforming the image pair to the MR atlas space and finally averaging the intensities for all transformed US images. If registration between modalities is accurate, then the constructed US template should be crisp. To evaluate the constructed templates, we compute two measures, Peak Signal-to-Noise Ratio (PSNR) with respect to our ground truth US template (Sect. 2.6) and the Variance of the image Laplacian (VAR), which provides an unbiased measure of sharpness [11]. Figure 4 shows that our method produces the sharpest template as measured by VAR and also has the highest PNSR. Furthermore, templates for our method have the same sharpness for any level of initial disorientation.

4   Conclusion

In this work, we proposed the LSTM spatial co-transformer, a deep learning-based method for group-wise registration of images to a standard pose.

We applied this to the challenging task of fetal MR/US brain image registration. Our method automatically coaligns brain images with a dual-modality spatio-temporal atlas, where future computational image analysis may be performed. Our results show that our method registers images more accurately than state-of-the-art similarity-based registration method "self-similarity context descriptors" [5]. Furthermore, it is able to robustly register highly misaligned images, where similarity-based will fail.

Acknowledgements. This work was supported by the Wellcome/EPSRC Centre for Medical Engineering [WT 203148/Z/16/Z], Wellcome Trust IEH Award [102431] and NVIDIA with the donation of a Titan Xp GPU.

References

1. Balakrishnan, G., Zhao, A., Sabuncu, M.R., Guttag, J., Dalca, A.V.: An unsupervised learning model for deformable medical image registration. In: CVPR (2018)
2. Cheng, X., Zhang, L., Zheng, Y.: Deep similarity learning for multimodal medical images. Comput. Meth. Biomech. Biomed. Eng. Imaging Vis. **6**(3), 248–252 (2018)
3. Cho, K., et al.: Learning phrase representations using RNN encoder-decoder for statistical machine translation. In: EMNLP, pp. 1724–1734 (2014)
4. Haber, E., Modersitzki, J.: Intensity gradient based registration and fusion of multi-modal images. In: Larsen, R., Nielsen, M., Sporring, J. (eds.) MICCAI 2006. LNCS, vol. 4191, pp. 726–733. Springer, Heidelberg (2006). https://doi.org/10.1007/11866763_89
5. Heinrich, M.P., Jenkinson, M., Papież, B.W., Brady, S.M., Schnabel, J.A.: Towards realtime multimodal fusion for image-guided interventions using self-similarities. In: Mori, K., Sakuma, I., Sato, Y., Barillot, C., Navab, N. (eds.) MICCAI 2013. LNCS, vol. 8149, pp. 187–194. Springer, Heidelberg (2013). https://doi.org/10.1007/978-3-642-40811-3_24
6. Jaderberg, M., Simonyan, K., Zisserman, A., Kavukcuoglu, K.: Spatial transformer networks. In: NIPS, pp. 2017–2025 (2015)
7. Kuklisova-Murgasova, M., et al.: Registration of 3D fetal brain US and MRI. In: MICCAI, pp. 667–674 (2012)
8. Lin, C.H., Lucey, S.: Inverse compositional spatial transformer networks. In: CVPR, pp. 2252–2260 (2017)
9. Mellor, M., Brady, M.: Phase mutual information as a similarity measure for registration. Med. Image Anal. **9**(4), 330–343 (2005). Functional Imaging and Modeling of the Heart - FIMH 2003
10. Ourselin, S., Roche, A., Subsol, G., Pennec, X., Ayache, N.: Reconstructing a 3D structure from serial histological sections. Image Vis. Comput. **19**(1), 25–31 (2001)
11. Pech-Pacheco, J.L., Cristobal, G., Chamorro-Martinez, J., Fernandez-Valdivia, J.: Diatom autofocusing in brightfield microscopy: a comparative study. ICPR **3**, 314–317 (2000)
12. Rivaz, H., Karimaghaloo, Z., Collins, D.L.: Self-similarity weighted mutual information: a new nonrigid image registration metric. Med. Image Anal. **18**(2), 343–358 (2014)

13. Rohé, M.-M., Datar, M., Heimann, T., Sermesant, M., Pennec, X.: SVF-Net: learning deformable image registration using shape matching. In: Descoteaux, M., Maier-Hein, L., Franz, A., Jannin, P., Collins, D.L., Duchesne, S. (eds.) MICCAI 2017. LNCS, vol. 10433, pp. 266–274. Springer, Cham (2017). https://doi.org/10.1007/978-3-319-66182-7_31

14. Serag, A., Aljabar, P., Ball, G., Counsell, S.J., Boardman, J.P., Rutherford, M.A., Edwards, A.D., Hajnal, J.V., Rueckert, D.: Construction of a consistent high-definition spatio-temporal atlas of the developing brain using adaptive Kernel regression. NeuroImage 59(3), 2255–2265 (2012)

15. Simonovsky, M., Gutiérrez-Becker, B., Mateus, D., Navab, N., Komodakis, N.: A deep metric for multimodal registration. In: MICCAI, pp. 10–18 (2016)

16. Wachinger, C., Navab, N.: Entropy and Laplacian images: structural representations for multi-modal registration. Med. Image Anal. 16(1), 1–17 (2012)

Automatic and Efficient Standard Plane Recognition in Fetal Ultrasound Images via Multi-scale Dense Networks

Peiyao Kong[1], Dong Ni[1], Siping Chen[1], Shengli Li[2],
Tianfu Wang[1(✉)], and Baiying Lei[1(✉)]

[1] National-Regional Key Technology Engineering Laboratory for Medical
Ultrasound, Guangdong Key Laboratory for Biomedical Measurement
and Ultrasound Imaging, School of Biomedical Engineering,
Shenzhen University, Shenzhen, China
{tfwang,leiby}@szu.edu.cn

[2] Department of Ultrasound, Affiliated Shenzhen Maternal and Child Healthcare
Hospital of Nanfang Medical University, Shenzhen, People's Republic of China

Abstract. The determination and interpretation of fetal standard planes (FSPs) in ultrasound examinations are the precondition and essential step for prenatal ultrasonography diagnosis. However, identifying multiple standard planes from ultrasound videos is a time-consuming and tedious task since there are only little differences between standard and non-standard planes in the adjacent scan frames. To address this challenge, we propose a general and efficient framework to detect several standard planes from ultrasound scan images or videos automatically. Specifically, a multi-scale dense networks (MSDNet) utilizing the multi-scale architecture and dense connection is exploited, which combines the fine level features from the shallow layers and coarse level features from the deep layers. Moreover, this MSDNet is resource efficient, and the cascade structure can adaptively select lightweight networks when test images are not complicated or computational resources limited. Experimental results based on our self-collected dataset demonstrate that the proposed method achieves a mean average precision (mAP) of 98.15% with half resources and double speeds in FSPs recognition task.

Keywords: Standard plane recognition · Prenatal ultrasound images
Resource efficient · Multi-scale dense networks

1 Introduction

Prenatal diagnosis of fetal abnormalities is quite important for both family and community. 2D ultrasonic examination is the most widely used prenatal diagnostic technique because of its low cost, radiation-free, and the ability to observe the fetus in real time. Prenatal ultrasonography generally involves image scanning, standard planes searching, structural observation, parameter measurement and diagnosis. The determination of standard planes is the precondition of structural observation, parameter measurement and final diagnosis [1], which is a crucial part of antenatal diagnosis.

© Springer Nature Switzerland AG 2018
A. Melbourne and R. Licandro et al. (Eds.): DATRA/PIPPI 2018, LNCS 11076, pp. 160–168, 2018.
https://doi.org/10.1007/978-3-030-00807-9_16

In fact, the judging of the standard plane requires deep knowledge and clinical experience [2]. In the underdeveloped areas, there are lack of the medical resources and experienced doctors. Also, standard plane screening is a time-consuming and laborious task. Therefore, it is of great significance to design an automatic standard plane recognition system, which not only improves the efficiency of prenatal ultrasound examination, but also reduces the burden of doctors.

Due to the continuity of the ultrasound scan images, there are only subtle difference between the standard image and the non-standard image from adjacent frames [3]. Compared with other imaging methods, ultrasound imaging is often affected by noise and artifacts such as shadowing, which results in poor imaging effect and affects the recognition accuracy [4]. As shown in Fig. 1, the first row is the standard plane images, and the second row is the non-standard plane images corresponding to different regions. It can be seen that it is quite difficult for non-professionals to accurately evaluate and distinguish FSPs images. Therefore, recognizing the standard image from ultrasound image automatically is a highly challenging task.

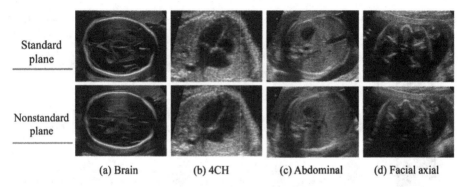

Fig. 1. Illustration of high similarity between standard and non-standard planes in ultrasound images. (a) brain; (b) four channel chamber (4CH); (c) abdominal; (d) facial axial.

In the recent years, deep learning is poised to reshape the feature of machine learning. Over the last decade, research on deep learning has made amazing achievements in many fields. The deep learning related methods has also been widely applied in analyzing medical images for prenatal analysis and diagnosis [5]. In fact, the core concept of deep learning is to learn data representations through increasing abstraction levels, which can learn more abstract and complex representations directly from the raw data. In addition, deep learning has been proved to have stronger applicability and better performance than traditional machine learning methods in the complex image recognition tasks [6]. For this reason, we mainly focus on deep network and representation in this study.

In order to ensure the portability of the algorithm and meet the diagnostic requirements in speed, our study focuses on the resource efficient planning model architecture. However, the previous deep learning studies on the standard image recognition task ignores the computing resources issue when designing the model, which makes the recognition quite slow [7]. Meanwhile, densenet has demonstrated the effectiveness of dense connections in the feature learning process in the related studies since its inception in 2017. For example, Huang et al. built a cascaded network MSDNet [8] based on the idea of dense connections and achieved good classification effect on the CIFAR dataset. Inspired by this, we exploit the MSDNet to build the FSPs recognition architecture. Experimental results on our collected in-house dataset show that our method is easier to mitigate the practical applications to achieve the real time detection in the clinical diagnosis.

2   Methodology

Figure 2 shows the architecture of our proposed method. There are four layers of our network. The specific model design of dense connection and cascade are described in the following sections.

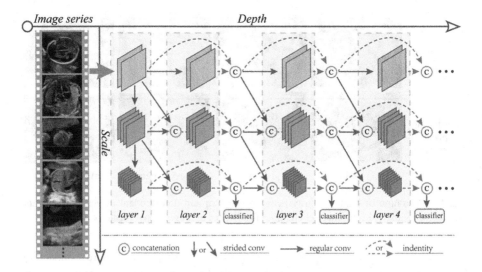

Fig. 2. The first four layers of our network. The horizontal coordinate represents the depth of the network, and the vertical coordinate represents the scale of the feature map. The dense connections across more than one layer are not explicitly drawn: they are implicit through recursive connections.

2.1   Network Architecture

The overall structure of the network is illustrated in Fig. 2. We use Fig. 3 to specify the dense connections in the model. The dense connection mode makes full use of the features with the low-complexity in the shallow layers, which allows the network to reuse and bypass the existing features of the previous layer and ensure high accuracy in later layers [9]. Moreover, dense connections also avoid gradient disappearance, which makes training faster and has less computational power for the same performance.

The network is designed as a cascade of layers that can be split or superimposed depending on the difficulty of different tasks. As can be seen from Fig. 2, there is a classifier designed between each layer and the second layer. This is designed for resource efficient, which enables the model output classification results at any layer of the network. This network adaptively chooses the deeper network for tough task and the shallow network for easy task. The performance of a classifier is located in the shallow layers of a general network, which is often poor due to the lack of coarse scale features. The multi-scale design in the architecture provides coarse scale and high-level feature representations that are amenable to classification.

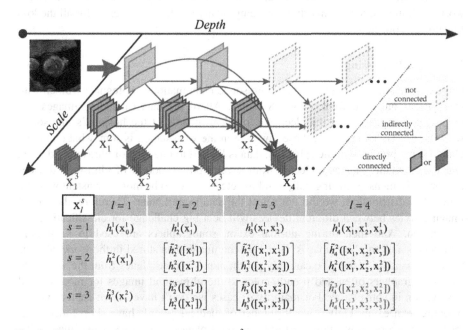

Fig. 3. Illustration of dense connections (e.g. x_4^3) and the list of output x_l^s of layer l in scale s.

The vertical connection on the first layer is designed to produce representations on all S scales. It can be thought as an S-layers convolutional network. As shown in Fig. 3, we use x_l^s to represent the output feature maps at layer l and scale s, and the original input is represented as x_0^1. Feature maps at coarser scales are obtained using the down-sampling method.

The feature maps x_l^s of each subsequent layers are a concatenation of all previous feature maps of scale s and $s-1$. At the bottom of Fig. 3, we have listed the formula for x_l^s of the first four layers. Here, we use $[\ldots]$ to represent concatenation operator, $h_l^s(.)$ is regular convolution, and $\tilde{h}_l^s(.)$ is stride convolution.

In order to test performance of any position in the network, a classifier is designed behind each layer. The classifiers use dense connection within coarsest scale S, such as the classifier at layer l uses all features $[x_1^s, \ldots, x_l^s]$. Afterwards, we identify the number of layers that are most suitable for our FSPs recognition task by relevant experiments about testing at any location of the model.

For all classifiers, we use cross entropy $L(f_k)$ as a loss function in training. The total cumulative loss functions is defined as

$$\mathcal{L}_{MSD} = \frac{1}{|\mathcal{D}|} \sum_{(x,y) \in \mathcal{D}} \sum_k w_k L(f_k) \tag{1}$$

where $\mathcal{D}$ represents the distribution of training dataset, w_k denotes the weight of the k-th classifier. Empirically, we find that using the same weight for all loss functions works well in practice. In this study, we empirically set the same weight for all the loss functions in our task.

2.2 Data Processing

Our dataset came from acquires 1499 ultrasound examinations of pregnant women with fetal gestational aged from 14 to 28 weeks. All of the data (including images and videos) is compiled from the electronic medical records of the hospital's ultrasound workstation. To some extent, those raw data in the workstation is somewhat cluttered. Unlike some previous studies [10, 11], data is limited to one type of ultrasound device. Our data contains images collected from several brand models of ultrasonic devices consist of Siemens, Samsung, GE, mindray, etc. In order to be more consistent with the actual data distribution, we did not select the data in particular. Therefore, the gap of imaging styles between different devices will be a big challenge for classification and recognition. And then during normal exam, sonographers are used to keep only important standard plane images. Hence all the image data stored in the workstation is basically standard plane. We can only get the non-standard planes from the video set. And sonographers often add pseudo-color to the ultrasound images for more careful observation in some cases. For majority of cases we don't have screen capture videos of entire fetal exam. Only a small number of medical records have short video fragments that record views adjacent to the standard planes. The same as the image data, the short videos also come from multiple branded devices. Each video was acquired from one patient and contained 17–48 frames. We used macro command to extract all their frames.

Because in this study we are only interested in structural information, we removed all color doppler ultrasound images by referring to the practice of ultrasound image data processing in other people's studies [10]. The images contains of doctor's marking and the split screen images showing multiple sections also be removed. In addition all pseudo-color images are converted to grayscale. According to the data situation, we combined our previous work and finally selected six standard plane on the advice of doctors. Finally, we have 22715 ultrasound images in our data set for FSPs recognition task. The detailed composition of data set is shown in Table 1. Moreover we divided the data into training set and test set in a ratio of 4:1.

Table 1. Data summary

Standard planes	Intro	ImageNum
Brain	Horizontal cross section of the thalamus	1840
4CH	Four-chamber view	2409
Abdominal	Standard abdominal view at stomach level	1687
Facial axial	Axial facial view at eyeball level	1585
Facial coronal	Coronal facial view of lips and nose	1959
Facial sagittal	Facial median sagittal view	1725
Others	Unmentioned standard views and non-standard planes	11510

3 Experimental Setting and Results

We implemented all of our models using PyTorch deep learning framework. The training was performed on a single Nvidia GTX Titan Xp, and 64G of RAM. In order to find out the best network depth (l) for our task. We firstly conducted the experiment of five-fold cross validation for different l. Therefore, we randomly divide all data into two parts in a ratio of 1:4, where the small part is used as the final test set and the large part is used for cross-validation. Afterwards, we set the network depth (l) to 15. The results of different depths is collected, and the train epochs is set as 300. We obtain the result of 5 verifications in each classifier, and the average accuracy of five tasks is shown in Fig. 4. In the broken line graph, it can be seen that the recognition accuracy has a significant upward trend at the beginning with the increase of network depth, and it becomes flattens out after the 7th layer. The broken line peaks at the tenth floor, then drops slightly and finally tends to be stable.

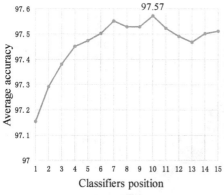

Table 2. Performance comparison of different networks

Model	FLOPs	ACC (%)	FPS
ResNet110	250.81 M	97.23	128.0
DenseNet100	292.23 M	97.64	137.7
Our ($l = 10$)	**148.01 M**	**98.26**	**226.9**

Fig. 4. The average accuracy of five cross validation by classifiers in different depth.

Based on the verification results in the previous step, we finally set the network depth as 10, take all the data used in the validation as the training set, training epochs is also set as 300. Table 2 shows the comparison of the computation amount, accuracy, and FSPs recognition speed (using frame rate measurements) of different networks. It can be seen that our model achieves nearly twice the speed and half the calculation compared with other networks. Our model obtains a recognition accuracy of 98.25%, which is the highest among all the listed models.

Considering that 'Others' class occupies a large proportion in the dataset compared with other classes, we measure the model performance using precision, recall and F1-score for each category. Table 3 shows the detailed test scores for all the standard planes. We can see that our method has achieved good performance in each category, and the average value of all three indicators is over 98%. In addition, the confusion matrix for this test is shown in Fig. 5. From the confusion matrix, we can observe the misclassification occurs between the standard surfaces and 'others' class because completely separating standard and non-standard planes is really a hard task.

Table 3. Recognition result (%)

Standard planes	Precision	Recall	F1-score	Images
4CH	98.76	99.38	99.07	481
Abdominal	96.41	95.55	95.98	337
FA	94.74	96.84	95.77	316
FC	98.42	95.40	96.88	391
Brain	100	100	100	368
FS	97.89	94.19	96.00	344
Others	98.45	99.22	98.83	2302
Avg/total	98.15	98.15	98.14	4539

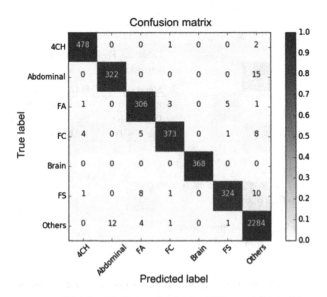

Fig. 5. Confusion matrix for MSD model

For the deep learning model, feature representation has a great impact on the recognition results. In order to more directly demonstrate the effectiveness of our network for FSPs recognition task, we use the t-SNE method [12] to visualize the test data and network feature maps. Specifically, for the original image, we convert the pixels of each image into a row vector and concatenate the values of all the sample vectors along the column dimension. We enter the pixel matrix and their labels into the t-SNE function. Similarly, the output feature vectors before linear layer of classifier are extracted, and t-SNE visualization is performed using the obtained representation form. The visualized results are illustrated in Fig. 6, where different colors in the diagram are used to represent data from different labels. One point in the figure represents one image sample, where a significantly larger number of purple marks represent 'others' classes. The left side of the figure is the distribution of the raw data in our testset, and the right side is the data distribution of the network classifier input feature maps (take $l = 10$ as an example). The mixed distribution of test data in the original domain shows that the class differences between FSPs and non-FSPs are very small, which makes our task challenging. We can clearly see that the deep representation after network processing makes the samples have obvious separability, which proves that the proposed model is very effective for FSPs recognition tasks.

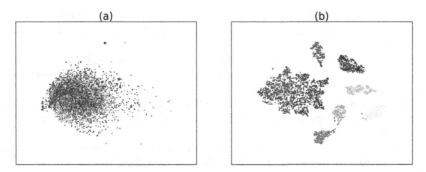

Fig. 6. t-SNE visualization results to illustrate the separability of deep representations in our model. (a) The raw test data distribution; (b) the distribution of data using our network.

4   Conclusion

In this paper, we propose an automatic and efficient FSPs recognition method based on MSDNet with powerful feature representation and efficient cascade design. We verify the effectiveness of our model on the ultrasound standard plane dataset for FSPs recognition task. We obtain the optimal number of network layers for our task through five-fold cross validation. Compared with other networks, the experimental results show that the proposed model achieves quite impressive performance (double speed and half calculations). Finally, through the analysis of multiple indicators, it is proved that our method achieves amazing performance in the recognition of each category. Furthermore, our approach is a general framework and can be extended to the other ultrasound standard planes recognition task. In future work, we will increase the variety of standard planes in the dataset and demonstrate the generalization ability of our model. Also, we will apply this algorithm to real-time detection in clinical practice.

References

1. Li, J., et al.: Automatic fetal head circumference measurement in ultrasound using random forest and fast ellipse fitting. IEEE J. Biomed. Health Inform. **22**, 215–223 (2018)
2. Cai, Y., Sharma, H., Chatelain, P., Noble, J.: SonoEyeNet: standardized fetal ultrasound plane detection informed by eye tracking. In: 2018 IEEE 15th International Symposium on Biomedical Imaging (ISBI 2018), pp. 1475–1478. IEEE (2018)
3. Chen, H., et al.: Automatic fetal ultrasound standard plane detection using knowledge transferred recurrent neural networks. In: Navab, N., Hornegger, J., Wells, W.M., Frangi, A. F. (eds.) MICCAI 2015. LNCS, vol. 9349, pp. 507–514. Springer, Cham (2015). https://doi.org/10.1007/978-3-319-24553-9_62
4. Milletari, F., et al.: Hough-CNN: deep learning for segmentation of deep brain regions in MRI and ultrasound. Comput. Vis. Image Underst. **164**, 92–102 (2017)
5. Shen, D., Wu, G., Suk, H.-I.: Deep learning in medical image analysis. Annu. Rev. Biomed. Eng. **19**, 221–248 (2017)
6. Litjens, G., et al.: A survey on deep learning in medical image analysis. Med. Image Anal. **42**, 60–88 (2017)
7. Wu, L., Cheng, J.-Z., Li, S., Lei, B., Wang, T., Ni, D.: FUIQA: fetal ultrasound image quality assessment with deep convolutional networks. IEEE Trans. Cybern. **47**, 1336–1349 (2017)
8. Huang, G., Chen, D., Li, T., Wu, F., van der Maaten, L., Weinberger, K.: Multi-scale dense networks for resource efficient image classification. In: International Conference on Learning Representations (2018)
9. Huang, G., Liu, Z., Weinberger, K.Q., van der Maaten, L.: Densely connected convolutional networks. In: Proceedings of the IEEE Conference on Computer Vision and Pattern Recognition, p. 3 (2017)
10. Baumgartner, C.F., et al.: SonoNet: real-time detection and localisation of fetal standard scan planes in freehand ultrasound. IEEE Trans. Med. Imaging **36**, 2204–2215 (2017)
11. Yu, Z., et al.: A deep convolutional neural network-based framework for automatic fetal facial standard plane recognition. IEEE J. Biomed. Health Inform. **22**, 874–885 (2018)
12. Donahue, J., et al.: DeCAF: a deep convolutional activation feature for generic visual recognition. In: International Conference on Machine Learning, pp. 647–655 (2014)

Paediatric Liver Segmentation for Low-Contrast CT Images

Mariusz Bajger[1,2], Gobert Lee[1,2(✉)], and Martin Caon[1,3]

[1] Medical Device Research Institute, Flinders University, Adelaide, Australia
{Mariusz.Bajger,Gobert.Lee,Martin.Caon}@flinders.edu.au
[2] College of Science and Engineering, Flinders University, Adelaide, Australia
[3] College of Nursing and Health Sciences, Flinders University, Adelaide, Australia

Abstract. CT images from combined PET-CT scanners are of low contrast. Automatic organ segmentation on these images are challenging. This paper proposed an adaptive kernel-based Statistical Region Merging (SRM) algorithm for paediatric liver segmentation in low contrast PET-CT images. The results are compared to that from the original SRM. The average dice index is 0.79 for SRM and 0.85 for the adaptive kernel-based SRM. In addition, the proposed method was successful in segmenting all 37 CT images while SRM failed in 5 images.

Keywords: Low contrast CT · PET-CT · Adaptive-kernel

1 Introduction

Children are sensitive to radiation dose. The use of ionizing radiation such as x-ray on children needs extra care. In some settings, segmenting of the liver from x-ray images may be required. Conventional CT images from dedicated CT scanners are typically involved due to high image quality but radiation dose is a concern. Combined PET-CT scanners generate CT images with lower radiation dose but the image has lower contrast. Automatic segmentation of organs from these low contrast CT images is challenging. A review of liver segmentation techniques can be found in [1,2].

A probabilistic atlas has been widely used for liver segmentation [3–6] and has produced good segmentation outcomes. In [3] Linguraru et al. have investigated the use of a probabilistic atlas for liver segmentation in low-contrast CT images. Based on a 20 patients' datasets (10 for training and 10 for testing) a Dice index of 88.2 ± 3.7 was achieved. The use of probabilistic atlas information can be augmented with other information. Li et al. [6] supplements the probabilistic atlas with primary liver shape and localization obtained from the PET scans. The probabilistic atlas was built using 60 CT studies from dedicated CT scanners. The PET-guided probabilistic atlas approach was applied on 35 PET-CT studies with a volume overlap percentage (VOP) of $92.9\% \pm 2.1$. In this approach, larger number of training data lead to improved segmentation results [3,6,7].

© Springer Nature Switzerland AG 2018
A. Melbourne and R. Licandro et al. (Eds.): DATRA/PIPPI 2018, LNCS 11076, pp. 169–178, 2018.
https://doi.org/10.1007/978-3-030-00807-9_17

In more recent studies, statistical shape model (SSM) has attracted a lot of interest [8–13]. A review of the statistical shape models for 3D medical image segmentation can be found in [14]. The results are promising but they also require large datasets for the SSM. For instance, in [13], 120 cases were used to develop the SSM. Annotation of the liver in the large training set is laborious.

The Statistical Region Merging (SRM) technique [15] is founded on Probability and Statistical theory and has been proposed for natural scene image segmentaion. The technique merges pixels into statistically homogenous regions (superpixels) to be regrouped into target objects/organs. Lee et al. [16] employed the SRM method [15] for multi-organ segmentation on non-contrast CT images. The technique has also been extended to 3D-SRM [17] for the spatial connectivity of volume CT data. Medical image segmentation based on the SRM method does not require large dataset for developing probabilistic atlas or statistical shape model. It does employ a prior knowledge of shape and location but primary segmentation of the liver on PET scans such as in [10] or the use of a simple model [18] suffices. In this paper, an adaptive kernel-based SRM (*kernel*-SRM) is proposed for segmentation of low contrast CT images. The method uses a kernel regressor and employs regional statistics. Results are compared with that of the SRM method.

2   Proposed Method

2.1   Adaptive *Kernel*-SRM

Consider a gray level intensity image of size $M \times N$

$$I : \{1, 2, \ldots, M\} \times \{1, 2, \ldots N\} \to [0, 255)$$

where $I(m, n) = f(m, n) + \epsilon$, with f being the true intensity value and ϵ the noise. The task is to estimate the unknown function f. In 1964 Nadaraya [19] (and also Watson [20]) proposed the following non-parametric estimator of the regression function

$$f(x, y) = E(I(X, Y)|(X, Y) = (x, y)), \tag{1}$$

where E denotes (conditional) expectation, and $((X, Y), I(X, Y))$ is the observed couple of random variables.

In order to estimate the regression function in Eq. (1), a non-parametric kernel-based estimator of Nadaraya-Watson type, which combines estimation and smoothing of the regression function, is commonly used. In this study, we consider a local version of the estimator defined for a given region in the image. The Nadaraya-Watson *local estimator* of the regression function $f(m, n)$, for a given region $\mathcal{R}$, can be defined as

$$\widehat{f}(m, n) = \sum_{(m_i, n_i) \in \mathcal{R}} w_i I(m_i, n_i), \tag{2}$$

$$w_i = \frac{K\left(I_i^{(m,n)}\right)}{\sum_{(m_i,n_i)\in\mathcal{R}} K\left(I_i^{(m,n)}\right)}, \tag{3}$$

$$I_i^{(m,n)} = \frac{I(m,n) - I(m_i,n_i)}{h_I}, \tag{4}$$

where $(m_i,n_i) \in M \times N$, K is a kernel function and h_I is the smoothing parameter for a given image I. Observe that (3) gives a weighted contribution from $I(m_i,n_i)$ to the estimated (true) value at (m_i,n_i).

As an example, consider the normal distribution $N_{\mu,\sigma}(m,n)$ with mean μ and standard deviation σ

$$N_{\mu,\sigma}(m,n) = \frac{1}{\sigma\sqrt{2\pi}} \exp\left(-\frac{1}{2}\left(\frac{I(m,n)-\mu}{\sigma}\right)^2\right). \tag{5}$$

The kernel is then defined as

$$K(I_i^{(m,n)}) = \frac{1}{\sigma\sqrt{2\pi}} \exp\left(-\frac{1}{2}\left(\frac{|I_i^{(m,n)}|-\mu}{\sigma}\right)^2\right) \tag{6}$$

where $|.|$ denotes absolute value.

From the definition of weights (3), one can observe that for a given image pixel the pixel's estimated (new) value will be most influenced by those local pixels whose intensities differ from the given one by the expected value of the intensity across the region. In other words, pixels having intensities very different from the given pixel intensity (with difference significantly bigger or smaller than the average intensity of the region) - noise pixels - will have little or no impact on the estimated intensity value (value of the regression function). Hence, assuming that the noise pixels have the distribution following the kernel function distribution the formula (2) can be effectively used to reduce noise in the image.

Using the notation in [15], the Statistical Region Merging (SRM) method allows merging of two regions R, R' if

$$|\bar{R} - \bar{R}'| \le \sqrt{b^2(R) + b^2(R')} \tag{7}$$

where

$$b(R) = g\sqrt{\frac{1}{2Q|R|}\ln\frac{2}{\delta}}, \tag{8}$$

$|.|$ denotes cardinality of a set, $\bar{R}$ denotes the average intensity across the region R, Q is a parameter which controls coarseness of the segmentation, $\delta = \frac{1}{6|I|^2}$ and g is the number of image intensity levels.

By incorporating an appropriate kernel function into the regional expectation $\bar{R}$ one can alleviate the effect of noise. Each time two pixels are considered for merging Eq. (2) is used to modify intensities in spatial neighbourhoods of these pixels. The radius for this neighbourhood was fixed to 2 pixels. This proposed method shall be called Adaptive Kernel-Based Statistical Region Merging method, and abbreviated as "kernel-SRM".

2.2   Determination of the Kernel Function

As described in the previous section, in order to successfully alleviate noise the kernel function corresponding to the noise distribution has to be determined. This is achieved by defining a structure-free region outside the human body on the CT image for image noise estimation. The primary variation of the image intensity in this region is due to noise. The histograms are built using the long-standing Sturges' rule [21] to estimate the number of bins $k = 1 + \log_2(n)$, where n is the number of data points.

The best fit probability density function was selected from the following range of distributions: Rayleigh, normal, Poisson, gamma and the generalized extreme value (GEV) distributions. In determining the most appropriate distribution, the Mean Square Error (MSE) was calculated for each fit and the distribution with the smallest MSE value was selected as the best fit.

3   Experiments and Results

3.1   Data

Thirty-seven paediatric liver CT images acquired from combined PET-CT scanner were included in this retrospective study. The images were de-identified and were obtained from a hospital in Sydney, Australia with ethics approval. The Siemens Emotion Duo scanner was used in acquiring the images with pixel size 0.98×0.98 mm and slice separation 0.34 mm. Ground truths of the liver regions were delineated by an expert in human anatomy and physiology (MC). CT images acquired from combined PET-CT scanners are of low image contrast and high noise level when compare with CT images acquired from dedicated CT scanners.

3.2   *Kernel*-SRM Segmentation

Image Pre-processing. Adaptive kernel-based segmentation is a computationally demanding process. To decrease the processing time, each CT image was automatically cropped to the area of the patient body. The CT images were then subsampled by 2 using the nearest-neighbour method to further reduce computational time.

Kernel Function/Image Noise Distribution Estimation. The kernel function (Sect. 2.2) of each CT image was estimated by automatically analysing the noise distribution in that image. In each image, the region comprising the top 120 rows of pixels across the full-width of the image is designated for noise distribution estimation. This region is outside the human body and is structure-free (anatomy-free). The histogram of the pixel intensities in this region was analysed (Sect. 2.2). Table 1 shows that in all but one case, the noise distribution was best estimated using normal distribution. For the remaining single case, the image

Table 1. Determination of the kernel function/image noise distribution estimation. The distributions Rayleigh, normal, Poisson, gamma and GEV were considered for the CT image noise estimation. The best fit with the smallest Mean Square Error (MSE) for individual CT are shown in below.

Index	Type	Param 1	Param 2	Param 3	Index	Type	Param 1	Param 2	Param 3
1	normal	25.01	9.60	–	20	normal	25.16	8.94	–
2	normal	24.47	9.96	–	21	normal	24.61	8.58	–
3	normal	25.10	9.72	–	22	normal	24.18	8.48	–
4	gev	−0.19	8.80	19.92	23	normal	24.58	8.98	–
5	normal	25.14	9.89	–	24	normal	24.73	8.57	–
6	normal	24.09	9.70	–	25	normal	24.66	8.93	–
7	normal	24.38	9.87	–	26	normal	24.09	8.50	–
8	normal	25.11	9.22	–	27	normal	24.96	8.04	–
9	normal	24.13	9.33	–	28	normal	24.38	8.35	–
10	normal	24.67	9.66	–	29	normal	23.94	7.82	–
11	normal	25.06	9.26	–	30	normal	25.06	8.11	–
12	normal	24.36	9.24	–	31	normal	24.52	8.89	–
13	normal	24.71	9.17	–	32	normal	24.10	8.53	–
14	normal	23.00	8.63	–	33	normal	24.99	8.45	–
15	normal	24.75	8.98	–	34	normal	24.58	8.36	–
16	normal	24.29	8.49	–	35	normal	24.23	8.37	–
17	normal	24.87	8.51	–	36	normal	24.63	8.87	–
18	normal	24.99	9.23	–	37	normal	24.90	8.39	–
19	normal	24.23	8.74	–					

noise has a generalized extreme value (GEV) distribution. In the proposed kernel-SRM method, the kernel function for each CT image was determined based on the estimated noise distribution of that image. Further analysis of these noise distributions shows that, for the normal distributions, the average of the mean parameter is 24.6 (std 0.45; range 23–25.2) and the average of the standard deviation parameter is 8.9 (std 0.6; range 7.8–9.9). One image has the generalized extreme value distribution with parameter $(\mu, \sigma, \xi) = (-0.19, 8.80, 19.92)$. Guided by these results, the normal (Gaussian) distribution with $\mu = 24$ and $\sigma = 9$ was selected as the kernel function.

Kernel Bandwidth Optimizing. The smoothing parameter h_I (Eq. 4), also known as the kernel bandwidth, was determined experimentally by searching over a wide range $[1, 30]$. Table 2 shows that the best segmentation result is achieved for $h_I = 3$. In addition, for $h_I \in \{2, 3, 4, 5\}$, the segmentation outcomes are similarly good with the average Dice index and average Hausdorff distance (in pixels) over all CT images being (0.84, 0.85, 0.84, 0.84) and (10.04, 8.77, 9.98, 10.48), respectively. This suggests that the performance of the proposed kernel-SRM is robust to small changes in the parameter h_I. The last column

Table 2. Optimization of the kernel bandwidth h_I. The parameter h_I was searched over the range [0.6, 30]. For each value of h_I, the average Dice index and the average Hausdorf value over all 37 kernel-SRM segmented livers are shown. The last column shows the number of CT images in which the kernel-SRM failed to segment the liver. The value of h_I producing the best results is boxed.

h_I value	Ave Dice	Ave Hausdorff	Failures
0.6	0.79	16.20	2
1	0.83	12.49	–
2	0.84	10.04	–
3	0.85	8.77	–
4	0.84	9.98	–
5	0.84	10.48	–
6	0.83	11.57	–
7	0.84	11.93	1
8	0.84	11.85	1
9	0.84	11.81	1
10	0.84	12.15	1
15	0.82	12.53	1
20	0.82	12.75	1
30	0.81	14.86	2

in Table 2 reports the number of CT images in which the proposed kernel-SRM method failed to generate a segmentation of the liver (Sect. 3.3).

3.3   Segmentation Representation and Evaluation Measures

As in the Statistical Region Merging (SRM) method in [15], through the employment of an appropriate value of the parameter Q (Eq. 8), the *kernel*-SRM was set to over-segmented the CT images, thereby, partitioned the images into statistically homogeneous regions (superpixels). These superpixels are non-overlapping. The union of these superpixels gives the exact image.

Over-Segmentation and Eligible Superpixels. In a perfect segmentation, the segmented liver would be ideally represented by a single superpixel. However, anatomical structures on CT images are not homogeneous. As such, the representation of the liver (target organ/tissue) is relaxed such that the segmented liver is represented by the union of one or more statistically homogeneous regions (superpixels). For a superpixel to be included in the segmented liver, over 50% of the superpixel must overlap with the ground truth which is unknown but can be estimated using different approaches such as the model-based approach [18]. In order to evaluate the performance of the proposed *kernel*-SRM against that of the SRM method without the interaction with ground truth estimated, the ground truth is used in this experiment. A superpixel satisfying this condition of >50% overlap is called an 'eligible' superpixel. Thus, the *kernel*-SRM/SRM segmented liver is the union of these 'eligible' superpixels. Though the number of the eligible superpixels in the segmented liver does not directly associate with the accuracy of the segmentation, when two segmentation outcomes are of similar accuracies, the one with a smaller number of eligible superpixels is of lower complexity and is a preferred solution. Figures 1a and b show two examples of the *kernel*-SRM segmentation outcomes. The ground truth was outlined in black and the eligible superpixel(s) that contributed to the *kernel*-SRM segmentation results are shown in patch(es) of color (false color for visualization). In the first example (Fig. 1a), only one eligible superpixel with a major (>50%) of the superpixel in the ground truth was found. In the second example (Fig. 1b), three eligible superpixels were found. Though two of them are small, over 50% of each the superpixel is in the ground truth. The *kernel*-SRM segmented liver is the union of these superpixels.

Failure - Resulting in Empty Set. If the liver is presented on a CT image but no eligible superpixels was found, this means that the liver segmentation on that image failed. The generated segmentation of liver is an empty set and no segmentation result was presented. Figures 1e and f show the SRM segmentation outcomes in two examples. The SRM statistically homogeneous regions (superpixels) were presented in false color for visualization. In Fig. 1e, less than 50% of the green superpixel overlap with the ground truth whereas in Fig. 1f, less than 50% of the purple superpixel overlap with the ground truth. Thus, the segmentation outputs are empty sets in both examples.

Segmentation Accuracy - Dice Index and Hausdorff Distance. For segmentation accuracy, Dice index and Hausdorff distance are measured on the segmentation outcome (union of the eligible superpixels), if eligible superpixel(s) is/are found. Dice index measures the agreement between the machine segmentation and the ground truth whereas Hausdorff distance measures the largest deviation between the two. If a segmentation outcome has no eligible superpixel, i.e. the segmentation failed, it follows that Dice index = 0 and the Hausdorff distance cannot be calculated.

3.4   Results and Discussions

Segmentation results of the proposed *kernel*-SRM and that of the original SRM are compared in this section. The results are generated with the kernel function a normal distribution with mean $\mu = 24$ and standard deviation $\sigma = 9$ (Sect. 3.2), an optimal bandwidth $h_I = 3$ (Sect. 3.2), and a g value of $g = 256$ for 256 grayscale level images and a Q value (Eq. 8) of $Q = 256$ determined empirically. Table 3 shows the average Dice index, average Hausdorff distance and the number of failures (Sect. 3.3). *Kernel*-SRM performs better than the SRM. The average

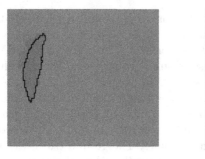
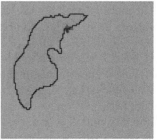

(a) Example 1: 1 eligible superpixel found (b) Example 2: 3 eligible superpixels found

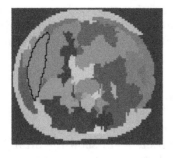
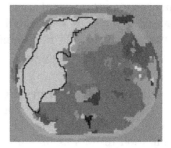

(c) Example 1:*Kernel*-SRM (proposed)   (d) Example 2:*Kernel*-SRM (proposed)

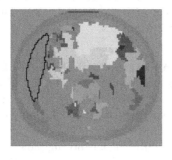
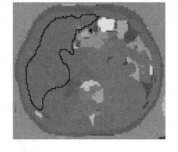

(e) Example 1:SRM   (f) Example 2:SRM

Fig. 1. Two Examples. The ground truth is delineation in black in all panels. Example 1 is presented in (a, c, e) and example 2 is presented in (b, d, f). Using the *kernel*-SRM, (a) 1 eligible superpixel (red) overlap with the liver was found in Example 1 and (b) 3 eligible superpixels (grey, green and dark blue) were found. The green and dark blue superpixels are small but over 50% is inside the ground truth, making them eligible. (c, d) *kernel*-SRM segmentation. The Dice index for (c) Example 1 is 0.88 and that for (d) Example 2 is 0.83. (e, f) SRM segmentation failed to produce any eligible superpixels in both examples as less than 50% of the green superpixel in example 1 and the purple superpixel in example 2 are inside the ground truth. Dice = 0 for both examples. (False color for visualization) (Color figure online)

Table 3. Comparison of SRM and *kernel*-SRM segmentation results.

	Ave Dice	Ave Hausdorff (in pixel)	Failure
SRM [15]	0.79	19.06[a]	14%(5/37)
Kernel-SRM (proposed)	0.85	8.77	0%(0/37)

[a]Excluding the 5 failure cases that Hausdorff distance cannot be calculated

Dice index and average Hausdorff distance over all 37 CTs were 0.79 and 19.06 for SRM and 0.85 and 8.77 for *kernel*-SRM, respectively. Moreover, SRM failed to segment (produced empty sets) in 5 cases while *kernel*-SRM was successful (no empty sets) in segmenting all images. Figures 2 and 3 show the detail of SRM and *kernel*-SRM comparisons in Dice index and Hausdorff distance, respectively. The five SRM failed examples are identified with Dice index = 0 in Fig. 2. Hausdorff distance cannot be calculated for the 5 failures and are shown with infinite lines in Fig. 3. Both Figs. 2 and 3 show that the *kernel*-SRM performs better in almost all cases.

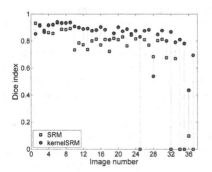
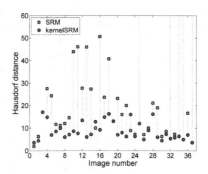

Fig. 2. Dice index - SRM vs. *kernel*-SRM liver segmentation results.

Fig. 3. Hausdorff distance (in pixel)- SRM vs. *kernel*-SRM results.

4   Conclusion

Segmentation of abdominal organs in low image contrast CT images generated from combined PET-CT scanners is challenging. This paper extended the well founded statistical region merging (SRM) method with a built-in kernel that handles the high level of image noise adaptively for every pair of regions to be considered for merging. Results showed that the proposed adaptive kernel-based statistical region merging (*kernel*-SRM) performs significantly better when compared with the original SRM method. The results, however, were found using a small dataset. Future work in validating the results with a larger dataset is required.

References

1. Gotra, A., Sivakumaran, L., et al.: Liver segmentation: indications, techniques and future directions. Insights Imag. **8**, 377–392 (2017)
2. Moghbel, M., Mashohor, S., et al.: Review of liver segmentation and computer assisted detection/diagnosis methods in computed tomography. Artif. Intell. Rev. (2017). https://doi.org/10.1007/s10462-017-9550-x
3. Linguraru, M.G., Li, Z., et al.: Automated liver segmentation using a normalized probabilistic atlas. In: Proceedings of SPIE, Medical Imaging, vol. 7262 (2009)
4. Linguraru, M.G., Sandberg, J.A., et al.: Atlas-based automated segmentation of spleen and liver using adaptive enhancement estimation. Med. Phys. **37**(2), 771–783 (2010)
5. Linguraru, M.G., Pura, J.A., et al.: Statistical 4D graphs for multi-organ abdominal segmentation from multiphase CT. Med. Image Anal. **16**, 904–914 (2012)
6. Li, C., Wang, X., et al.: Automated PET-guided liver segmentation from low-contrast CT volumes using probabilistic atlas. CMPB **107**, 164–174 (2012)
7. Zhou, X., et al.: Constructing a probabilistic model for automated liver region segmentation using non-contrast X-ray torso CT images. In: Larsen, R., Nielsen, M., Sporring, J. (eds.) MICCAI 2006. LNCS, vol. 4191, pp. 856–863. Springer, Heidelberg (2006). https://doi.org/10.1007/11866763_105
8. Okada, T., Linguraru, M.G., et al.: Abdominal multi-organ segmentation from CT images using conditional shape-location and unsupervised intensity priors. Med. Image Anal. **26**, 1–18 (2015)
9. Saito, A., Nawano, S., Shimizu, A.: Joint optimization of segmentation and shape prior from level-set-based statistical shape model, and its application to the automated segmentation of abdominal organs. Med. Image Anal. **28**, 46–65 (2016)
10. Li, G., Chen, X., et al.: Automatic liver segmentation based on shape constraints and deformable graph cut in CT images. IEEE TIP **14**(12), 5315–5329 (2015)
11. Shi, C., Cheng, Y., et al.: A hierarchical local region-based sparse shape composition for liver segmentation in CT scans. Pattern Recognit. **50**, 88–106 (2016)
12. Wang, X., Zheng, Y., et al.: Liver segmentation from CT images using a sparse priori statistical shape model (SP-SSM). PLoS ONE **12**(10), e0185249 (2017)
13. Tomoshige, S., Oost, E., et al.: A conditional statistical shape model with integrated error estimation of the conditions: application to live segmentation in non-contrast CT images. Med. Image Anal. **18**, 130–142 (2014)
14. Heimann, T., Meinzer, H.-P.: Statistical shape models for 3D medical image segmentation: a review. Med. Image Anal. **13**, 543–563 (2009)
15. Nock, R., Nielsen, F.: Statistical region merging. IEEE Trans. Pattern Anal. Mach. Intell. **26**(11), 1452–1458 (2004)
16. Lee, G., Bajger, M., Caon, M.: Multi-organ segmentation of CT images using statistical region merging. In: Proceedings of the 9th IASTED International Conference on Biomedical Engineering, pp. 199–206 (2012)
17. Bajger, M., Lee, G., Caon, M.: 3D segmentation for multi-organs in CT images. Electron. Lett. Comput. Vis. Image Anal. **12**(2), 13–27 (2013)
18. Sedlar, J., Bajger, M., et al.: Model-guided segmentation of liver in CT and PET-CT images of child patients based on statistical region merging. In: Proceedings of the DICTA, pp. 156–163 (2016)
19. Nadaraya, E.A.: On estimating regression. Theory Probab. Appl. **10**, 186–190 (1964)
20. Watson, G.S.: Smooth regression analysis. Sankhya Ser. A **26**, 101–116 (1964)
21. Sturges, H.A.: The choice of a class interval. J. Am. Stat. Assoc. **21**, 65–66 (1926)

Author Index

Printed in the United States
By Bookmasters